UNDERSTANDING THE ANTIOXIDANT CONTROVERSY

UNDERSTANDING THE ANTIOXIDANT CONTROVERSY

Scrutinizing the "Fountain of Youth"

PAUL E. MILBURY AND ALICE C. RICHER

616.07
M638

The Praeger Series on Contemporary Health and Living
Julie Silver, Series Editor

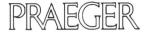

Westport, Connecticut
London

Library of Congress Cataloging-in-Publication Data

Milbury, Paul E., 1950–
    Understanding the antioxidant controversy : scrutinizing the "fountain of youth" /
    Paul E. Milbury and Alice C. Richer.
        p. ; cm. – (The Praeger series on contemporary health and living, ISSN 1932–8079)
        Includes bibliographical references and index.
        ISBN 978–0–275–99376–4 (alk. paper)
        1. Antioxidants–Health aspects–United States.   2. Antioxidants industry–United States.
3. Dietary supplements–United States.   4. Functional foods–United States.   I. Richer, Alice C.
II. Title.   III. Series.
        [DNLM: 1. Antioxidants–therapeutic use–United States.   2. Antioxidants–adverse
effects–United States.   3. Antioxidants–metabolism–United States.   4. Dietary
Supplements–United States.   QV 325 M638u 2008]
    RB170.M52   2008
    616.07–dc22   2007029900

British Library Cataloguing in Publication Data is available.

Library of Congress Catalog Card Number: 2007029900
ISBN-13: 978–0–275–99376–4
ISSN: 1932–8079

First published in 2008

Praeger Publishers, 88 Post Road West, Westport, CT 06881
An imprint of Greenwood Publishing Group, Inc.
www.praeger.com

Printed in the United States of America

The paper used in this book complies with the
Permanent Paper Standard issued by the National
Information Standards Organization (Z39.48–1984).

10 9 8 7 6 5 4 3 2 1

CONTENTS

Series Foreword by Julie Silver   vii

Acknowledgments   ix

Preface   xi

1. The Perception of Antioxidants in America   1

2. The Science of Nutrition   15

3. Antioxidants and the Redox Biology of Life   31

4. What Does Research Show?   51

5. The Antioxidants of Life   81

6. Making Sense of It All   103

Appendices

    A: Dietary Reference Intakes   118

    B: Antioxidants–Dietary Reference Intakes   125

    C: Resources   129

Glossary   133

Notes   147

Index   171

SERIES FOREWORD

For years I have wanted to read a book exactly like *Understanding the Antioxidant Controversy*. Patients ask me daily what supplements they should and shouldn't take. They are clearly intelligent and informed, and they have heard different things about supplements from the media. Indeed, it's not the media's fault that the message is confusing (though beware of sensationalism with regard to this topic), as the authors of this book, Paul Milbury and Alice Richer, point out "antioxidants appear to have a Jekyll and Hyde personality." A book by experts who are able to evaluate the scientific data and report on it clearly and without bias is exactly what we have needed for years. Milbury and Richer did just that when they teamed up to write *Understanding the Antioxidant Controversy*. This book is an excellent evidence-based guide for consumers, health care providers, policymakers, health reporters, and scientists who are studying vitamins, minerals, and supplements. Fortunately for those of us who need to better understand the antioxidant controversy, Milbury and Richer wrote not only a book based on the science currently available on this topic but also a fascinating guide that includes many wonderful anecdotes and stories to go along with the important facts and statistics.

Julie Silver, M.D.
Assistant Professor
Harvard Medical School
Department of Physical Medicine and Rehabilitation

ACKNOWLEDGMENTS

I would like to thank my family for their love, support, and patience as I wrote this book. I also want to thank my friends and cheering section—Cathy Weiner and Gloria Marsh. Cathy, you always believe in me and words can never thank you enough for being such a great friend. Gloria, what can I say? It's your turn.

Thanks to my great coauthor Paul—I enjoyed working with you and your invaluable knowledge and guidance made this book a reality. Most of all I wish to thank Julie Silver without whom this book would not have been possible. Julie, your help and confidence means more to me than words can ever say. Last of all I want to thank God, who has blessed and continues to bless my life so much.—*ACR*

In a busy and complicated life it is always good to have organized folks among those you work with. I am extremely grateful to my coauthor Alice for her hard work and organizational skills that were invaluable in bringing this book to fruition.—*PEM*

PREFACE

Antioxidants—the new Fountain of Youth? Media reports and dietary supplement manufacturers would seem to support this assumption. But antioxidant nutrients and their mechanisms of action within the human body are far more complex than most of us realize. In 1957, the research scientist Denham Harmon proposed the free radical theory of aging. His theory proposed that the consequence of aging was the result of "attacks" upon our body tissues by radicals due to oxidative stresses. These oxidative stresses, the result of pollution, cigarette smoke, UV rays from the sun, and (even worse) normal metabolism caused disease and aging.

Studies suggest that vitamins C and E, polyphenols, and the nutrient selenium could slow down disease progression and postpone the aging process. Needless to say, media sources have been quick to report the possible benefits of antioxidants and dietary supplement sales have increased dramatically. But antioxidants appear to have a Jekyll and Hyde personality. While some research shows positive benefits, others show no effects or, even worse, negative results. One study, using high-dose vitamin E supplements, showed all causes of death actually increased when this antioxidant was taken.

Americans are aging and health care costs have been spiraling out of control in recent years. Increasing numbers of Americans are distrustful of conventional medicine and turning to alternative therapies. Special interest groups and dietary supplement manufacturers successfully lobbied Congress and strict guidelines for dietary supplements were drastically relaxed in 1994. The FDA, charged with the safety of Americans, is unable to do this job in large part because of the Dietary Supplement Health and Education Act of 1994, also known as DSHEA. Yet many Americans and health care professionals are unaware that dietary supplements are largely unregulated. Controversy surrounds antioxidants and both consumer and healthcare professional find they are confused about what to do.

The goal of this book is to clear up some of this confusion and outline the best course of action where antioxidants are concerned. We will look at the state of the science regarding antioxidants and consumer attitudes toward complementary and alternative therapies. We will delve into how many Americans take supplements and who they turn to for information. We will explore the science of nutrition and the history of food and drug regulations. The complex science of redox biology (where antioxidants live) will be explained and a synopsis of antioxidant study results will be laid out. Each antioxidant will be explained, recommendations given, and the reader will be alerted to the benefits and dangers of dietary supplements, especially when taken without medical supervision. Last, but not least, we will provide what we believe is the best way to include antioxidants into every day life.

Understanding the Antioxidant Controversy will educate both health professional and consumers and should prove to be a valuable resource when dealing with the subject of antioxidants and health.

1

THE PERCEPTION OF ANTIOXIDANTS IN AMERICA

The average American has come to perceive antioxidants as the first line of defense against aging and chronic disease. Even though scientific studies report conflicting results and do not yet provide specific guidelines, dietary supplement use in the United States, which includes antioxidants, continues to rise. Concern over dietary supplement usage and safety issues due to unquestioned consumer confidence in supplement effectiveness and safety is growing as well. This has prompted many health agencies—such as the National Academy of Sciences, Institute of Medicine (IOM), National Institute of Health (NIH), and the World Health Organization (WHO)—to study vitamin, mineral, and antioxidant efficacy and use, subsequently issuing statements that establish interventions, consumer education programs, and recommendations.

Improvements in living conditions, food supply, and medical care have increased life expectancy in the United States to its current 77.9 year average.[1] As a nation we are an aging population, with those aged 65 years and older increasing from 12 to 36 million between 1950 and 2004.[2] The Centers for Disease Control and Prevention (CDC) *The State of Aging and Health in America 2007 Report* estimates the number of Americans aged 65 and older will double to over 71 million (see Figure 1.1), or about 20 percent of the entire population, by 2030.[3] This aging population, which is three to five times more likely to require health care services for chronic health issues and projected to represent about 25 percent of our nation's health care expenditures,[4] is starting to take a more proactive approach toward their health. The result is increased use of complementary and alternative medicine (CAM) therapies, which includes dietary and antioxidant supplements.[5]

The Food and Drug Administration (FDA) estimates there are over 29,000 dietary supplements already in the market with approximately 1,000 new products developed annually.[6] The *Nutrition Business Journal* (NBJ), a research and consulting company analyzing nutrition and health markets, estimated 2005 U.S. dietary supplement sales at $20.9 billion (a $2.1 billion increase from 2003). Thirty-four percent of total supplement sales, or $7.1 billion, was

Figure 1.1
Population by Age

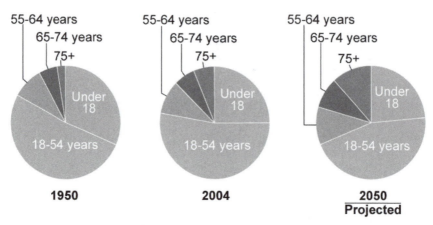

Source: Centers for Disease Control and Prevention, National Center for Health Statistics, *Health, United States, 2005*, figure 2.

spent on vitamins and minerals and represented an increase of an estimated $3 billion dollars since 1995.[7]

The most recent supplement category to emerge is functional foods, also called nutraceuticals. The term "functional food" describes a food category that usually includes foods high in antioxidant content. While there is currently no formal regulatory definition associated with the term, functional food is defined by the IOM as "any food or food ingredient that may provide a health benefit beyond the traditional nutrients it contains."[8] Apples and blueberries are examples of "functional foods" that possess (in theory) disease-preventive qualities. Even salt, fortified with iodine as of 1924 to prevent goiters, is considered a functional food. The term "nutraceutical" encompasses functional foods but also includes supplements and, more recently, cosmoceuticals—cosmetics to which food extracts or ingredients are added. Beverages with added vitamins not inherently present, for example, are considered nutraceuticals. Corporate goals to meet consumer demand has led to including ingredients containing "healthy" properties—such as antioxidants, carotenoids, isoflavones—into their products resulting in many foods reaching the market with dramatic changes to their fundamental nutritional composition. With the addition of a "healthy" ingredient(s), marketing claims are sometimes made that a food product will provide a specific health benefit to the consumer. As a result, 65 percent of Americans reported purchasing functional foods/nutraceuticals in 2005 and spent an estimated $36 billion on them. Functional food/nutraceutical sales are expected to grow at a rapid rate[9] largely due to the passage of the Dietary Supplement Health and Education Act of 1994 (DSHEA) that allowed companies to market supplements, herbals, and functional foods without government approval.[10] This legislation defined the types of products to be regulated as dietary supplements and established regulatory procedures for making health claims on supplement labels. In particular, claims that generally deal with prevention, treatment, or cure of disease are considered drug claims and cannot be included on food product labels. But the FDA does allow claims to be made about the effects a food or ingredient has on the structure or function of the body without any review or approval.

Expanding knowledge of genetics, proteomics (the study of proteins in the body in relation to genetics), and molecular biology are leading to new theories of promoting diet to treat or prevent illness. The science of nutrigenomics is the most recent nutrition frontier. Nutrigenomics studies diet and lifestyle choices and their effect on individual genetic risk factors. The hope for the future is that, based on genetic markers of disease risk, diet can be tailored to the individual that will, in theory, reduce or prevent the manifestation of disease.

Rapid changes are occurring in the food and nutrition markets and most grocery shoppers report they attempt to improve and/or manage chronic illness using foods. The health and food industries, and even pet food manufacturers, are embracing the antioxidant phenomenon and condition-specific, risk-reducing products are being introduced at a rapid rate. While Americans have been blessed with a longer average life expectancy, longevity has not come without a price. Individuals over the age of 55 tend to exhibit more severe health issues, chronic disease incidence, and increased dependence on prescription drugs. Our national health care costs, doubling between 1993 and 2004, are projected to gradually overwhelm our economy.[11] Because older consumers are more likely to be focused on health issues and possess extra disposable income, they have become very attractive marketing targets. With Americans looking to improve health, extend life, decrease medical costs, and take matters into their own hands, dietary supplement manufacturers and marketers see a golden opportunity. While antioxidants have been promoted as the twenty-first century's solution for improved health and eternal youth, are they really the answer?

THE HEALTH OF OUR NATION

As a nation we have made significant progress in controlling many diseases and reducing mortality rates through public health programs, research, education, health care, and advances in medical technology. Vaccination and food fortification programs have virtually eliminated some of the most devastating diseases, such as polio, typhoid, and rickets, common in previous generations. But chronic diseases associated with aging and longer life expectancies, especially among racial and ethnic groups, have brought new challenges. Americans reporting fair or poor health due to chronic health conditions increases significantly with age.[12]

In 2004, Americans spent more money on health care than any other country, spending an average of about $6,280 per person.[13] While most

Americans have private health insurance, health costs have risen dramatically and the insurance industry has increasingly shifted health care costs onto the consumer, mostly through out-of-pocket expenses. Between 1997 and 2002, consumer out-of-pocket health care expenses increased from 17 to 20 percent. Prescription drug costs represented about 23 percent of total out-of-pocket expenses for those aged 55 to 64. Added to increasing health care costs is the burden of the uninsured. In 2003, 17 percent of Americans under the age of 65 years, in a minority group, or with incomes below or at poverty level were uninsured.[14]

Dissatisfied with conventional health care and concerned about pharmaceutical side effects, increasing numbers of patients are being drawn to the use of CAM therapies. CAM therapies include health care practices and products that are not usually prescribed by conventional medical practitioners. They include acupuncture, Aruveyda, chiropractic and massage therapies, special diets, and vitamin/mineral/antioxidant and megavitamin therapies. In 1994, 40 percent of the general public reported CAM use and Americans spent between $36 billion to $47 billion on CAM therapies in 1997—mostly out-of-pocket.[15] The majority of CAM users are educated, affluent, and were between the ages of 30 and 49. Their expressed dissatisfaction with conventional medicines' ability to treat chronic illness was cited as the main reason they turned to CAM therapies.[16]

Increases in life expectancy, chronic disease incidence, uninsured and out-of-pocket health care expenses, and a changing attitude toward conventional medicine with a trend toward self-care, finds American consumers more focused on disease prevention and management than ever before. The perceived benefits that antioxidant supplements represent—improved disease management, decreased effects of aging, and lowering of health care expenses—has become very appealing to the average American.

There is no doubt that media attention about the health benefits of dietary antioxidants and CAM therapies influence their use. A survey by the American Dietetic Association (ADA) in 2000 found that most Americans become educated about food, nutrition, and health via media sources. Table 1.1 shows that only 11 percent of Americans learn about nutrition and health from a physician as opposed to 48 percent who learn about it from television.[17]

But media sources have often lacked a complete scientific understanding and confusion and misinformation often is the result. Sixty-eight percent of respondents in a National Health Council Survey agreed with the statement, "When reporting medical and health news, the media often contradict themselves, so I don't know what to believe." A Rodale Press survey found that most consumers find stories about vitamins, supplements, and nutrition to be the most confusing of all reported health stories. As a result, the International Information Council (IFIC) Foundation and the Harvard School of Public Health convened an advisory group in 2003 to examine health and media communication, issuing guidelines for more responsible health communication practices by the media.[18]

Table 1.1
Information Sources from which Americans Learn about Food, Nutrition, and Health Topics

Information Source	Percent (%) of Americans
Television	48%
Magazines	47%
Newspapers	18%
Books	12%
Family/Friends	11%
Doctor	11%
Internet	6%
Radio	5%

Source: Data from American Dietetic Association, "Nutrition and You: Trends 2000: What Do Americans Think, Need, Expect?" *Journal of American Dietetic Association* 100 no. 6 (2000): 626–627.

But even though Americans often express confusion, dietary supplement use continues to increase. Sales of vitamin A increased by 100 percent, vitamin C by 42 percent, and vitamin E by 178 percent between 1987 and 2000.[19] Negative press reports can also affect vitamin use, often with more lasting effects. Sales of vitamin E after 2000 offer a striking illustration. A meta-analysis study published in 2004[20] found negative health outcomes when large doses of vitamin E supplements were taken. The negative press surrounding this study resulted in an almost 40 percent decline in vitamin E sales, which still have not rebounded to previous levels.[21]

Attempts to estimate conclusive supplement use in the United States is elusive. Surveys analyzing American eating habits began in 1935, but comprehensive studies of health and nutrition status began with the passage of the National Health Survey Act of 1956. This legislation provided a way to evaluate current trends of illness and disability in the United States on a continuous basis. The survey that resulted from this Act was called the National Health Interview Survey (NHIS) and is still conducted today by the National Center for Health Statistics (NCHS). The United States Department of Agriculture (USDA), NCHS, and the FDA fund the most reliable and scientific surveys. Survey results are analyzed and the information is used to develop public health policies.

Studies about diet and nutrition habits are traditionally retrospective studies—a look back at past food intake by a statistical representation of the population using interviews or questionnaires. This preferred study method is less costly and labor intensive and can be applied to large populations. Accuracy of the data depends on questionnaire design, skill of the interviewer, adequate size and representative population sample, response rate, and accuracy of data collection and analysis. Data collection and survey formats have evolved over time. Food recalls, varying between twenty-four hours and seven days, have been used with questions about supplements and medicines added over time. The most informative nutrition and health surveys are the NHIS, Nationwide Food Consumption Survey (NFCS), the Continuing Survey of Food Intakes by Individuals (CSFII), the National Health Examination Surveys (NHES), The Ten State Survey, and the Health and Nutrition Examination Survey (NHANES). Other studies, such as the Diet and Health Knowledge Survey (DHKS) and Health and Diet Survey, provide information about consumer food awareness, attitudes, practices, and expenditures. In an effort to establish a diet/nutrition link and reduce costs and duplication efforts, the NHES and CSFII were incorporated into the NHANES.

NHANES is one of the most comprehensive and objective national surveys conducted today, studying a representative sample of the U.S. population using direct interview, physical examination, and medical record reviews to analyze health, lifestyle, and diet. All other surveys rely on self-reported information. NHANES surveys were completed between 1971 and 1975 (NHANES I), 1976 and 1980 (NHANES II), and 1982 and 1984 (HHANES–Hispanic population). The 1988 to 1994 NHANES III included more specific questions about dietary supplement use for the first time. Beginning in 1999, the Continuous NHANES was implemented and smaller representative population samples began to be studied annually. Since most individuals tend to underreport what they eat and data is dependent on individual memory, random errors can be significant. Therefore, data collected from the National Eating Trends Survey, directed by the business company NPD Group, is combined periodically into the NHANES to keep the database as accurate as possible.

The Continuous NHANES (1999 to 2000) found about 52 percent of adults took a dietary supplement over the past year. This showed a steady increase in use from 40 percent reported in the NHANES III, 35 percent in the NHANES II, and 23 percent in the NHANES I. Characteristics of reported supplement users, shown in   Table 1.2, revealed that the majority were women, over the age of 60, white, educated, physically active, and already practicing healthy lifestyle habits. The most popular supplements consumed were multivitamins/multiminerals (35%) followed by vitamin E (12.7%), vitamin C (12.4%), and calcium (10.4%; 25.5% if taken as an antacid).[22] Of the 1900 reported supplements taken by consumers, 47 percent contained at least one antioxidant (see Figure 1.2).[23]

Other scientific studies, summarized in Figure 1.3, such as the NHIS, CSFII, and the American Dietetic Association (ADA) Nutrition and You Trends: 2000, found similar results.[24]

In general, the NHANES results have been regarded as a conservative estimate of dietary supplement use in America. Despite safeguards, the general opinion of the IOM is that this data underreports actual intakes and may be preconceived in some cases. But the NHANES still provides a snapshot of nutrient intakes by the U.S. population and provides a way of assessing needs. Other surveys find supplement use is higher than the NHANES reports. The 2002 Health and Diet Survey reported 73 percent of Americans took

Table 1.2
Characteristics and Percent (%) of Antioxidant Dietary Supplement Users

Characteristic	Any supplement	MVI/MM	Vt. A	Vt. C	Vt. E	Selenium
Total	52.0%	35.0%	1.3%	12.4%	12.7%	1.1%
Male	46.9%	31.7%	1.2%	12.2%	11.7%	1.1%
Female	56.7%	38.0%	1.5%	12.6%	13.5%	1.0%
Age						
20–39	43.3%	30.4%	1.0%	8.9%	4.4%	0.4%
40–59	56.1%	37.8%	1.5%	13.7%	15.3%	1.6%
≥60	63.3%	39.8%	1.8%	17.3%	25.3%	1.6%
Non-Hispanic White	58.2%	39.8%	N.D.	14.7%	15.5%	N.D.
Non-Hispanic Black	36.0%	23.0%	N.D.	5.1%	5.4%	N.D.
Mexican American	33.3%	20.5%	N.D.	4.5%	4.9%	N.D.
<High school education	34.7%	21.4%	N.D.	5.7%	7.5%	N.D.
High school education	48.4%	30.5%	N.D.	9.9%	11.2%	N.D.
>High school education	62.2%	43.9%	N.D.	16.9%	16.0%	N.D.
BMI			N.D.			N.D.
<25.0	56.8%	39.5%		13.1%	12.9%	
25–30	51.7%	34.3%		13.1%	14.0%	
≥30.0	46.3%	30.1%		10.8%	10.7%	
Exercise			N.D.			N.D.
none	42.5%	26.4%		10.2%	10.2%	
moderate	58.9%	40.6%		13.7%	15.3%	
vigorous	58.5%	41.3%		14.0%	13.7%	
Health			N.D.			N.D.
Excellent	54.9%	38.8%		13.5%	13.2%	
Good	49.6%	31.6%		12.2%	12.4%	
Fair/poor	46.7%	28.5%		8.7%	11.6%	
Cigarette use			N.D.			N.D.
never	52.2%	36.0%		12.8%	13.9%	
former	61.2%	41.6%		14.8%	16.7%	
current	43.0%	26.6%		9.2%	6.3%	
Beer/wine/spirits			N.D.			N.D.
Never	47–53%	31–34%		10–12%	11–14%	
1–4 times/mth	52–59%	35–40%		12–16%	12–16%	
≥5 times/mth	50–72%	36–51%		14–23%	11–24%	

MVI = multivitamin; MM = multimineral; N.D. = No data
Source: Adapted from Kathy Radimer, et al., "Dietary Supplement Use by US Adults: Data from the National Health and Nutrition Examination Survey, 1999–2000," *American Journal of Epidemiology* 160 (2004): 339–349.

supplements. Of those acknowledged supplement users, 85 percent took a multivitamin/multimineral, 77 percent took a single ingredient vitamin, and 42 percent took other supplements.[25] Food marketing, consumer magazines, and Internet quick polls estimate use to be even higher. A *Prevention Magazine* survey in 2001 found 85 percent of adults queried reported taking a daily dietary supplement over the past year.[26] Although much smaller sample sizes

Figure 1.2
Number of Supplements Containing Antioxidants (NHANES 1999–2000)

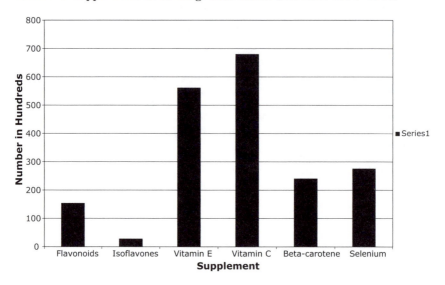

Figure 1.3
Percent of Americans Using Dietary Supplements

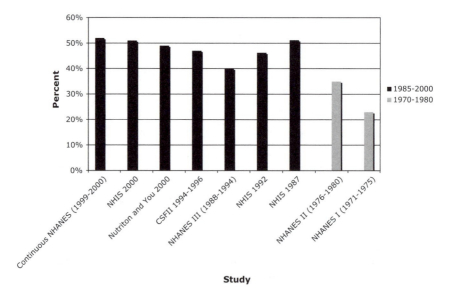

and self-reporting methods were used for these surveys, they shed some insight into consumer attitude and behavior regarding dietary supplements.

Many Americans assume dietary supplements are closely regulated by the government. Because of this belief, nearly two-thirds of consumers believe supplements are safe to take.[27] Between 50 percent and 72 percent taking daily supplements did so to treat or prevent illness, to feel better, or to live longer. Fifty-three percent of those taking functional foods/nutraceuticals believe they offer benefits drugs do not and 56 percent felt they were comparable to drugs but with fewer side effects. Ninety-five percent were satisfied with the supplements they took. Not surprisingly, only 33 percent took them on the advice of their physician.[28]

A recent Health and Wellness Trend Report by the National Marketing Institute (NMI) found consumers associate antioxidant supplements with cancer prevention (32%), immune function (23%), and heart health (17%). Adults with medical conditions were more likely to take a dietary supplement. Nearly 81 percent of breast cancer survivors, with a high risk for recurrence, reported taking regular supplements and men with coronary artery disease, hypercholesterolemia, and hypertension were more likely to take vitamin E supplements as well.[29] Even more alarming is that most regular supplement and functional food/nutraceutical users, particularly those taking prescription medications, never tell their physician they are taking them because they believe the doctor knows little about them or may be biased against their use. Many supplement users have indicated they would continue to take supplements even if scientific studies proved them to be ineffective.[30]

THE MEDICAL COMMUNITY AND SUPPLEMENTS

Many health care professionals find they are just as confused about supplements as the general public. Because of the many uncertainties surrounding the effectiveness and safety of supplements, most physicians err on the side of caution. A few studies about physician health and treatment practices shed some insight on how physicians handle the topic of dietary supplements with their patients. As a group, physicians generally have a healthier lifestyle and lower mortality rate than the general public. Physicians with healthy habits are more likely to discuss preventive health behaviors with their patients, than those who do not, which in turn appears to influence counseling practices.[31]

Not many studies have investigated physician attitude toward dietary supplement and CAM therapies. A literature search turns up two studies worthy of note. The first examines physician attitude toward CAM therapies. This study found most physicians, the majority being women and younger than 46 years old, were open-minded and would refer their patients to a CAM practitioner if they were affiliated with their group practice site (about 44%). But most physicians did not discuss CAM with their patients unless the patient broached the subject first and few discussed possible harmful outcomes. The majority of physicians were familiar with biofeedback, chiropractic and massage therapies, acupuncture, relaxation, and megavitamin treatments. They were least familiar with homeopathy and naturopathy treatments. While many felt CAM therapies can present a safety threat to the public, they also perceive that offering CAM therapies will attract patients to their practices and offer promising new forms of treatment. It is noted that by 1998, 64 percent of medical schools incorporated some form of CAM education into their curricula, indicating future physicians will be much better informed about CAM therapies and medicines.[32]

The second study investigated vitamin-mineral use by female physicians. As noted previously, physicians' personal health habits influence patient counseling habits. Data from the Women's Physicians' Health Study (WPHS) found 50 percent of women physicians took multivitamin/multimineral supplements occasionally and 35.5 percent took them daily. Of note is that those physicians with a medical condition—such as heart disease or diabetes—were more likely to take a daily dietary supplement, most often vitamin E. It is extrapolated that these physicians are more likely to recommend dietary supplement use to their patients than those who do not use supplements.[33]

SUPPLEMENT SAFETY

So just how safe are the supplements that have become a regular part of some Americans daily diet? The jury is still out. As mentioned before, Americans believe that dietary supplements are evaluated as strictly as pharmaceutical drugs and are safe to take, not realizing they are regulated as food and therefore not as stringently controlled. DSHEA defined what a dietary supplement is, increased public access to supplements, and established different safety requirements from pharmaceutical drugs. But DSHEA's major flaw has been lack of oversight and the curtailing of FDAs authority to remove harmful products from the marketplace. Manufacturers have sole responsibility in determining supplement effectiveness and safety and are not mandated to report adverse events. The FDA only learns about adverse events through voluntary consumer complaints, poison-control centers, and surveillance programs such as MedWatch. Many consumer advocacy groups, such as Public Citizen, are critical of the FDA and are fighting for more stringent regulations and oversight. With the exception of the United States, most countries regulate supplements and functional foods/nutraceuticals as drugs with strict testing and regulation *before* they are sold to consumers.

Data from the 2002 Health and Diet Survey found 4 percent of supplement users experienced at least one adverse event after taking a dietary supplement. The majority of those experiencing adverse events were between the ages of 35 to 54, female, and had taken either a multivitamin/multimineral, calcium, vitamin C, iron, vitamin B, vitamin E, and/or assorted botanicals. A 1998 survey of eleven U.S. poison-control centers learned about one-third of all reported adverse supplement events were associated with severe symptoms,

Table 1.3
Adverse Events Reported after Dietary Supplement Use

Most Common Symptoms	Percent (%)
Heart Problems/Chest Pain	12.5%
Abdominal Pain	8.4%
Headache	7.7%
Rashes	6.7%
Allergy/Reactions	6.0%
Nausea	5.1%
Blood Pressure problems	4.7%
Diarrhea	4.5%
Cramping/Muscle Aches	4.4%
Dizziness/Fainting	3.1%
Sleep Problems	2.8%
Less-frequently reported symptoms	29.7%

Source: Adapted from Babgaleh Timbo, et al., "Dietary Supplements in a National Survey: Prevalence of Use and Reports of Adverse Events," *Journal of American Dietetic Association* 106, no. 12 (2006): 1971.

such as seizures, coma, myocardial infarction, arrhythmia, coagulation disorders, hepatic diagnosis, anaphylaxis, and death. Table 1.3 provides a synopsis of the most common symptoms associated with these adverse events. Of those consumers who experienced an adverse reaction, either 90 percent stopped taking the supplement, 48 percent saw their physician, 25 percent reported the event to a health authority, 12 percent went to the emergency room, or 9 percent complained to the manufacturer or place of purchase.[34]

Of note is that 31 percent of those reporting adverse events took the supplement while also taking a prescription drug and 21 percent of them were taking the supplement on the advice of a physician/health professional. Thirteen percent took a supplement instead of a prescribed drug to treat/prevent a health condition and only 7 percent of them discussed this substitution with their physician/health professional.[35]

Because an increasing number of people are affected by adverse dietary supplement reactions (still low overall), public safety concerns expressed by patient advocacy groups and health care professionals has risen. Subsequently, the Dietary Supplement and Nonprescription Drug Consumer Protection Act was signed into law in December 2006. This law will require dietary supplement manufacturers to notify the FDA of all serious adverse events reported and also require a reporting telephone number on all dietary supplement labels.

SUPPLEMENT EFFICACY

There is evidence that use of multivitamin-mineral supplements is generally not harmful and could measurably improve health (i.e., heart disease, cancer, immune function, and cataracts), particularly among the young, the elderly, those with chronic illnesses, low-income populations, and overweight patients.[36] But, it is known that high levels of many of the minerals (i.e., iron, zinc, copper, selenium) and some fat-soluble vitamins (i.e., vitamin A and β-carotene) can be toxic. However toxic levels can be avoided when multivitamin/mineral supplements are taken properly.

Relatively few clinical trials with high-quality methods have been carried out on vitamin/mineral use in chronic disease that are generalizable to the U.S. population. Of those studies using high-quality methods, few have shown unequivocal beneficial effects. Two large trials testing lung cancer prevention with β-carotene supplements actually experienced an increase in lung cancer incidence and death in smokers and male asbestos workers. Other studies have not shown a reduction in cancer occurrence. The Carotene and Retinol Efficacy Trial (CARET) resulted in increased stroke and cardiovascular disease risk in women smokers.[37] Vitamin A intake, not yet studied individually, when combined with β-carotene, increased lung cancer and cardiovascular disease death rates. Vitamin A, when combined with zinc, did not prevent cancer occurrences. One study found a decrease in cardiovascular deaths when vitamin E was taken. Yet other trials using vitamin E supplementation have yielded inconclusive results and vitamin E use has been associated with increased bleeding, subarachnoid hemorrhage, and hemorrhagic strokes.[38]

It is a fair assumption that more hard data is needed to determine dietary supplement benefits and risks. The U.S. supplement industry is largely unregulated and supplement/functional food/nutraceutical use continues to increase. Most supplement users are healthy and at low risk for nutritional inadequacies. Worldwide trials of vitamin C, vitamin E, selenium, β-carotene, and other carotenoids were reviewed in 2000 by a panel appointed by the IOM of the National Academies of Science, which was charged with establishing Dietary Reference Intakes (DRIs) for these antioxidants.[39] The panel concluded, as of 2000, there was insufficient evidence to support claims that taking mega doses of dietary antioxidants, such as selenium, vitamins C and E, or carotenoids (including β-carotene) prevents chronic diseases. Hypernutrition (excess nutrient intake) and public safety issues are fast becoming emerging concerns.

More stringent government interventions are currently being put into place, such as the Dietary Supplement and Nonprescription Drug Consumer Protection Act. The National Center for Complementary and Alternative Medicine (NCCAM), established in 1992, is focused on encouraging more scientific studies, training of CAM researchers, and provision of reliable and accurate information to both the public and health care professional. The Nutrient Databank System, maintained by the USDA, has expanded to now include data about flavonoid, carotenoid, and isoflavone composition of foods. Additional databases listing dietary supplement ingredients are also in development.

The NIH concluded in their 2006 State of the Science Multivitamin/Mineral Supplements and Chronic Disease conference[40] that:

1. More accurate information is needed about dietary supplement use in the population and study methods need to be improved.
2. Dietary supplement databases need to be built with ingredient information and regular updates.
3. Effective communication methods to disseminate scientific information to the public are needed.
4. Dietary supplement and medication interactions must be studied.
5. Population segments, previously underrepresented and at risk for chronic disease, need to be studied.
6. New biomedical sciences, such as nutrigenomics, need to be studied and techniques applied to observational and randomized, controlled, clinical studies.
7. Efficacy and safety of individual vitamins, minerals and vitamin/mineral combinations need to be studied more rigorously.

As we explore antioxidants more in-depth, keep in mind that in general, the evidence available to us today does not recommend for or against the use of antioxidant dietary supplements to prevent chronic disease and decrease the effects of the aging process. Americans are taking a calculated risk when using dietary supplements, antioxidants, and functional foods/nutraceuticals.

2

THE SCIENCE OF NUTRITION

There is no question that antioxidants are intricately involved with the metabolic processes of human life. Many metabolic reactions require them and dire consequences can sometimes result in their absence. But while they look promising in the lab, supplementation in humans has proven to be much more complicated. Media hype—quick to tout antioxidant benefits—and increasing dietary supplement sales (thanks in part to relaxed regulations and a growing consumer trend toward self-care) has created controversy and a quagmire. The public, while confused by information that often conflicts, trusts dietary supplements to be beneficial, safe, and effective. Health professionals and research scientists have mixed conflicting opinions with some promoting antioxidant supplements as an "insurance policy" regardless of study results while others discourage use of them at all.

The relationship between the foods we eat and our health has been recognized for thousands of years. For most of human existence, just securing enough food for survival was paramount. Foods were eaten when and where they were found without any thought to nutritional value. Available foods were highly dependent on climate and environment, and choices were certainly not determined by the proximity of a fast food restaurant. As early man developed tribal and social behaviors, food customs and restrictions evolved that were based on superstition (for example, eating the flesh of aggressive, strong animals bestowed courage and strength). These customs became classified within religious rules and beliefs and were often driven by anecdotal observations of shamans or healers, who were also spiritual leaders, and carried forward to subsequent generations. But as medical science began to evolve so did our experience with food-based remedies. Historical records report the Roman statesman Cato the Censor (234–149 B.C.) believed eating cabbage restored and preserved health.[1] Night blindness, caused by a vitamin A deficiency, was recorded as early as 1500 B.C. by the early Egyptians who cured it with an extract of ox liver (high in vitamin A) applied to the eyes.[2] Greek historian

Herodotus (484–425 B.C.) was one of the first to observe a connection between sunshine and vitamin D. As he visited battlefields after a conflict, he noticed that Persian skulls were much more fragile than Greek skulls, which were strong. The fact that the Greeks wore no head coverings, unlike the Persians who wore turbans, led to the premise that exposure of the head to the sun made the skull stronger.[3] Hippocrates, long regarded the "Father of Medicine," prescribed myrtle, barley mush, apples, dates, linseed, wheat flour, beans, millet, eggs, water from crab apples, and "milk of asses taken hot" to treat illnesses, and he also prescribed liver to cure night blindness. While Hippocrates realized there was a connection between food and health, his knowledge of what food components were responsible for health effects was still incomplete.[4]

The earliest record of a nutrition experiment can be found in the Old Testament of the Bible in the Book of Daniel. Daniel and his Jewish brethren were allowed to eat pulses (vegetables) and water while all the other young men in the King's court drank wine and ate the royal delicacies. After ten days Daniel and his colleagues "looked healthier and better nourished than any of the young men who ate the royal food."[5] The seventeenth century marked the beginning of modern science and by the 1700s medical and nutrition research, although still in their infancy, were firmly established.

Vitamin discoveries came to the forefront in 1740 when a physician for the British navy, James Lind, carried out the first controlled nutrition experiment and "discovered" the treatment for scurvy.[6] This hemorrhagic disease, a very common and deadly disease (especially among sailors), was a well-known scourge and killed an estimated 2 million sailors between 1500 and 1800.[7] The French explorer Jacques Cartier recorded the effects of scurvy during his exploration of Canada in 1535 with 110 of his men. Traveling with the St. Lawrence Iroquois Indians, a number of his men and some of the Indian guides became ill with scurvy during the winter months. As the end of winter neared, no more than ten of his men were well and twenty-five had died. After speaking with the Iroquois Chief's son, Domagaya, an infusion from the needles of the white cedar tree annedda (rich in vitamin C) were given to the men and the crew was cured.[8]

Dr. Lind treated scurvy victims with seven different substances, finding lemon and lime juices cured the illness. While this documents the unofficial discovery of vitamin C (vitamin C would not be officially "discovered" until 1932), the importance of Dr. Lind's discovery was not fully realized and more than forty years would pass before lime juice would become a staple on British naval ships (hence the nickname British Limeys).[9] Also during the 1700s Antoine Lavoisier, known as the "Father of Nutrition," became the first to document the interrelationship between food and energy metabolism in the body. Carbohydrates, proteins, and fats were later determined to be important food components essential for health. But it wasn't until Jean Baptiste Andre' Dumas (1800–1884), who discovered that food possessed other equally important nutrients, that nutrition research moved forward.[10]

Earnest study of the science of nutrition began in the twentieth century. In 1911, Casimir Funk was the first to identify vitamins. Establishing them as essential nutrients, he named them vitamines (believing they were made of amines containing nitrogen; the name was later changed to vitamin (1920) when it was discovered that most vitamins did not contain nitrogen).[11] The research of Elmer Vernon McCollum and associates during the 1900s led to the discovery of many essential vitamins and minerals needed in the human diet. Some of McCollum's more important research discovered vitamins A and B, and explored the relationship between diet, sunshine, and rickets. Vitamin D was subsequently discovered and widespread supplementation of human diets with vitamin D-rich cod liver oil was initiated in the United States, representing the first food fortification program. The common and disabling diseases of the time—beri-beri (thiamine deficiency), scurvy (vitamin C deficiency), rickets (vitamin D deficiency), pellagra (niacin deficiency), and kwashiorkor (protein calorie malnutrition)—long attributed to infections, were found to be nutrient deficiencies and represented a major public health breakthrough leading to national food fortification programs. Research began to prove good nutrition did make a difference in health.[12]

Between 1940 and 1950, four fat-soluble and eleven water-soluble vitamins had been identified as essential elements for humans and are listed in Table 2.1. During this same period, mineral ash (the noncombustible fraction of foods) was also found to be essential. Twenty-one different mineral elements, listed in Table 2.2, were established as essential and classified as macronutrients and micronutrients. From 1950 until the present, the focus of nutrition research began to shift from discovery to identification of causal relationships between nutrition and health and disease.[13]

VITAMINS AND MINERALS

The individual cells in our bodies operate much like factories. The essential building blocks of enzymes, as well as essential cofactors and energy availability, are required for cells to operate properly and ensure survival of the human body. As we now know, vitamins and minerals are essential for life-sustaining chemical reactions to occur. An essential nutrient is defined as "one that must be provided to the organism by food because it cannot be synthesized by the body at a rate sufficient to meet its needs."[14] Essential nutrients vary between the different species. When critical vitamins and minerals needed for healthy cell maintenance, growth, and development are removed from the diet, deficiency symptoms eventually become apparent. Depending on body stores, symptoms of these deficiencies can occur relatively rapidly or take months to develop in humans.

Vitamins are defined as "organic substances, needed in very small amounts, that perform a specific metabolic function and must be provided in the diet of the animal."[15] They work as catalysts and substrates in metabolic reactions and some vitamins also function as cofactors for enzymes, assisting them to

Table 2.1
Discovery of Vitamins

Vitamin	Discovery	Other Common Names
Water-soluble		
Thiamin (Vt. B_1)	1921	Antineuritic factor
		Antiberiberi factor
Inositol (no longer a vt.)	1928	Muscle sugar
Choline	1930	
Ascorbic Acid (Vt. C)	1932	Antiscorbutic factor
Riboflavin (Vt. B_2)	1932	Yellow enzyme
		Vt. G
		Lactoflavin, Ovoflavin
Panthothenic Acid	1933	Animal Protein Factor (APF)
		Pantothenol
Pyridoxine (Vt. B_6)	1934	Pyridoxic acid
		Pyridoxal, Pyridoxamine
Biotin	1935	Anti-egg-white injury factor
		Vitamin H
Niacin	1936	Nicotinic Acid
		Niacinamide
Folic Acid	1945	Folacin
		Vitamin M
		Factor U
Cobalamin (Vt. B_{12})	1948	Cyanocobalamin
		Antipernicious anemia factor
		Erythrocyte maturation factor
Fat-soluble		
Vitamin A	1915	Retinoic Acid
		Retinal, Retinol
Vitamin D	1918	Cholecalciferol
		Ergocalciferol
		Antirachitic factor
Vitamin E	1922	Tocopherol
		Antisterility factor
Vitamin K	1934	Phytylquinone
		Antihemorrhagic factor

Source: Adapted from Guthrie, *Introductory Nutrition,* 3rd ed., 1975, 198–199.

function. Vitamins are classified into two categories: fat-soluble and water-soluble. The fat-soluble vitamins are absorbed through the intestinal tract with the aid of dietary fats. Because they are stored by the body, foods containing them do not have to be eaten daily and deficiencies are slow to develop. The water-soluble vitamins dissolve easily in water and deficiencies develop rapidly because they are excreted from the body if taken in excess. Vitamins are usually obtained from food sources, but a few can actually be manufactured within the body. Vitamin K, for example, is synthesized by microorganisms in

Table 2.2
Essential Minerals

Classification	Element
Macronutrients:	Calcium
	Chlorine
	Magnesium
	Phosphorus
	Potassium
	Sodium
	Sulfur
Micronutrients:	Chromium
	Cobalt
	Copper
	Fluorine
	Iodine
	Iron
	Manganese
	Molybdenum
	Nickel
	Selenium
	Silicon
	Tin
	Vanadium
	Zinc
Trace Minerals:	Arsenic
	Barium
	Bromine
	Cadmium
	Strontium
Trace Contaminants:	Aluminum
	Antimony
	Bismuth
	Boron
	Gallium
	Gold
	Lead
	Lithium
	Mercury
	Silver

Source: Adapted from Guthrie, *Introductory Nutrition,* 3rd ed., 1975, 105.

the intestine, vitamin D by the skin from ultraviolet rays in sunlight, and niacin is converted from the amino acid tryptophan available in meat. Another group of essential nutrients, vitamin precursors, are chemically related to vitamins. Vitamin precursors (also known as provitamins) cannot be used until converted by the body to its active form. One example is beta-carotene, the vitamin precursor of vitamin A.[16]

Essential dietary minerals are chemical elements that assist in the regulation of fluid balance, muscle contractions, and nerve impulses. They are classified as macronutrients, micronutrients, trace minerals, and trace contaminants. Macronutrients are those minerals needed in amounts of at least 100 mg per day or more. Micronutrients are needed in amounts no higher than a few milligrams per day. Trace minerals may be essential, but no conclusive evidence has established this. Trace contaminants are minerals found in the environment that are ingested unintentionally and have no known need. Minerals are absorbed through the intestine and the body usually regulates mineral stores to keep them in balance. As a rule, excess minerals are excreted, but some drugs, medical illnesses, and dehydration can interfere with mineral balance and result in deficiencies, toxicity, and sometimes even death.[17]

ANTIOXIDANTS

Dietary antioxidants are compounds that (in theory) reduce oxidative damage to the body by free radicals. Free radicals are highly reactive chemicals that have the potential to attack critical molecules within the body, changing their chemical structures and affecting their function. Oxidative stress is defined as an imbalance between the levels of various reactive oxygen species (molecules or compounds that react easily and can cause cell damage, such as superoxide, hydrogen peroxide, hydroxyl radicals) and the ability of the body's natural protective mechanisms to control and cope with these reactive compounds before they cause damage to cells or cellular processes. Oxidative stress-induced damage and the consequent alterations to metabolism and biologic function are hypothesized to cause many chronic diseases and contribute to the natural aging process. The most well-known antioxidants are vitamins C, E, selenium, carotenoids (i.e., beta-carotene, lutein, and lycopene), and phytochemicals known as flavonoids. Antioxidant vitamins, precursors, and minerals are thought to counteract oxidative damage and some have been used as additives for many years by food chemists or chefs to prevent or delay food spoilage. For example, vitamins C or E are used to prevent or delay the enzymatic browning reaction (oxidation) of apples, peaches, and potatoes once they are peeled and/or cut-up and thus exposed to air.

In 2000, the Institute of Medicine (IOM) defined the term antioxidant and published antioxidant recommendations. The Food and Nutrition Board of the IOM defined a dietary antioxidant as "a substance in foods that significantly decreases the adverse effects of reactive species, such as reactive oxygen and nitrogen species, on normal physiological function in humans."[18] Vitamin C is considered an antioxidant because of its ability to render harmful free radical reactions harmless. Vitamin E is believed to work as a chain-breaking antioxidant by preventing lipid peroxidation, which is the interaction between free radicals and cell membrane lipids that can cause cell damage. Selenium functions as an oxidant defense enzyme. Carotenoids are important primarily because they convert into vitamin A when needed and are theorized to have possible antioxidant activity. However, other than their known roles in the human body, the role of antioxidants in disease prevention still has not been determined.

Polyphenols, a large group of naturally occurring plant compounds, contain flavanoids (also known as bioflavonoids that include isoflavones, anthocyanins, catechins, epicatechin), tannins, lignins, and stilbenes. As the name implies, polyphenols have at least two phenolic rings in their structures. They are included among the important antioxidants because, *in vitro* at least, their structures provide them with potent antioxidant activity. As will be discussed later, their *in vivo* antioxidant function may have more to do with their ability to modulate cell metabolism than in direct quenching of radicals. Some polyphenols are thought to improve cardiovascular health by increasing capillary strength and some are thought to decrease the risk of diseases such as arthritis and cancer. Green tea extract and resveratrol (found in grapes and red wine) are currently two of the more popular polyphenols.

Bioflavonoids, one grouping of polyphenols, were first identified in the 1930s and designated as vitamin P, though very quickly the validity of calling them vitamins was questioned because clear deficiency symptoms were not evident. By 1950, vitamin P was changed to the classification bioflavonoids. Between 1950 and 1990, many more polyphenols were discovered but no substantial evidence of their essential role in nutrition has been presented, nor have definitive guidelines for their use yet been established.[19]

RDA, RNI, AND DRI

With scientific studies validating the importance of various substances, compounds, and nutrients for good health, the emerging public health challenge was to ensure that daily nutrient requirements were met. Nutrient standards were developed and became known as the Recommended Dietary Allowance (RDA). The RDAs became the "yardstick" used to develop public health nutrition programs and policies. The National Research Council issued the first set of RDAs for energy, protein, vitamins, and minerals in 1941. By 1989, the RDAs had been revised nine times and had expanded from eight nutrients to twenty-seven. In 1938, the Canadian Council on Nutrition issued the Dietary Standard for Canada, later renamed the Recommended Nutrient Intake (RNI) in 1983. Revised a total of four times, the focus of the RNIs since 1990 has been on chronic disease reduction.[20]

RDA and RNI values have been used as the gold standard to evaluate diet adequacy in individuals and for populations when developing food fortification programs, food labels, and nutrition education programs. However, the U.S. and Canadian nutrient standards differed in definition, revisions, and interpretation leading to some confusion. Because of these differences, the Food and Nutrition Board of the IOM in 1994 set out to establish recommended nutrient intakes to replace and expand upon the RDAs and RNIs. In 2006 the IOM published a common set of scientifically grounded reference values for chronic disease prevention in healthy populations known as the Dietary Reference Intakes (DRIs). The DRIs replace both the RDAs and RNIs and represent a change in current nutrition practices.[21] The new DRI standards for vitamins and minerals can be found in Appendix A.

The new DRIs, summarized in Table 2.3, are divided into four nutrient-based reference values: Estimated Average Requirement (EAR), Recommended Dietary Allowance (RDA), Adequate Intake (AI), and Tolerable Upper Intake Level (UL). These values are also divided up into different life stage groups and are for use with healthy populations only—those with illnesses or deficiencies are not included. The DRIs provide a reasonable estimate of nutrient requirements to provide adequacy and prevent excess intake. But even these revisions have drawbacks. The EARs are based on a small sample of individuals with approximated and uncertain requirements, assume individual requirements follow a normal distribution curve, and extrapolate values for all population groups. Thus it remains difficult to ascertain specific individual diet requirements with total certainty. In actual clinical practice it is essential to consider other factors as part of a comprehensive nutrition assessment when formulating individual diet recommendations.[22]

DIETARY SUPPLEMENT REGULATIONS

Regulation of dietary supplements has had a long and sometimes controversial history. Most Americans assume dietary supplements are as tightly regulated as OTC and prescription medications are. But with the passage of the Dietary Supplement Health and Education Act of 1994 (DSHEA), dietary supplement controls were relaxed. Supplement manufacturers are no longer required to provide data supporting safety as required for both OTC and prescription drugs. In order to understand the evolution of current regulations, it is insightful to explore the history of food and drug regulations.

In the 1800s contaminated, diluted, and counterfeit drugs were common. Medicines containing morphine, heroin, cocaine, and opium were sold without oversight or disclosure and unsuspecting consumers sometimes experienced devastating results. Growing concern in the United States in the 1800s over drug and food safety came to a head around the 1840s. The newly formed American Medical Association (AMA) and pharmacists joined together to establish legislation that would enforce drug purity and potency standards, known as the Import and Drugs Act of 1848. It was an important first step in ensuring public safety. As the United States moved toward becoming an industrialized nation, it became necessary to provide food to the increasing city populations from distant areas. At this point in time, cows were not yet tested for tuberculosis, milk was not pasteurized, and the only refrigerant available to prevent food spoilage was ice—all commonplace public health safety controls we take for granted today. By 1862 reports of problems with food preservation and use of chemical preservatives were growing. The Pure Food Movement, pushed by food industry members, set the stage for legislation to protect the public

Table 2.3
DRI Definitions and Life Stage Groups

Estimated Average Requirement (EAR)	The average daily nutrient intake level that is estimated to meet the requirements of half of the healthy individuals in a particular life stage and gender group.
Recommended Dietary Allowance (RDA)	The average daily dietary nutrient intake level that is sufficient to meet the nutrient requirements of nearly all (97–98%) healthy individuals in a particular life stage and gender group.
Adequate Intake (AI)	The recommended average daily intake level based on observed or experimentally determined approximations or estimates of nutrient intake by a group (or groups) of apparently healthy people that are assumed to be adequate; used when an RDA cannot be determined.
Tolerable Upper Intake Level (UL)	The highest average daily nutrient intake level that is likely to pose no risk of adverse health effects to almost all individuals in the general population. As intake increases above the UL, the potential risk of adverse effects may increase.
Life Stage Groups	DRI values are assigned to life stage groups that correspond to the different stages of the human lifespan. They are: • Infancy: 1 to 6 months and 7 to 12 months • Toddlers: age 1 to 3 • Early Childhood: age 4 to 8 • Puberty/Adolescence: age 9 to 13/age 14 to 18 (male & female) • Young Adulthood/Middle age: age 19 to 30 (male & female)/ age 31 to 50 (male & female) • Adulthood/Older Adults: age 51 to 70 (male & female)/ over 70 years (male & female) • Pregnancy • Lactation

Source: Adapted from Food and Nutrition Board, Institute of Medicine of the National Academies, "Dietary Reference Intakes," 2006, 8–16.

against adulterated foods. Food was adulterated when ingredients were added that presented unknown risks or a significant or unreasonable risk for injury or illness. With growing fraud in the food and patent medicine industries and the publication of Upton Sinclair's *The Jungle*, which exposed the unsafe and unsanitary conditions in the Chicago meat packing industry, efforts by the U.S. government to ensure public safety intensified. The Pure Food and Drug Act became law on June 30, 1906. Broad authority was given to the federal government to protect the public from adulterated and mislabeled drugs and foods. The government agency, Bureau of Chemistry, administered this law and built the foundation upon which many of our current food and drug laws exist today. The Bureau of Chemistry later reorganized and became known as the Food and Drug Administration (FDA) in 1931. Although the Bureau of Chemistry was given legal authority against manufacturers of illegal products, they were unable to enforce punishment against false label claims.[23] Emerging technologies in production and marketing of food and drugs, along with the economic hardships experienced in the 1920s, made the 1906 law obsolete by the 1930s. On June 25, 1938, after much debate and conflict, the Federal Food, Drug, and Cosmetic Act (FD&C Act) was signed into law. For the first time drug and food manufacturers were held accountable for the safety and claims they made about their products. The FDA was given authority to punish violators and new drug applications were required for all new drugs, resulting in intense scrutiny for safety issues, before being allowed on the market. A product was regarded as an unapproved drug if claims were made that it treated or prevented a disease (a disease claim).[24]

In 1903 Dr. Harvey Wiley, then head of the Bureau of Chemistry, established safety standards for some chemical preservatives through the volunteer efforts of the "Poison Squad." The Poison Squad, a group of young men who volunteered to eat only foods that had been treated with measured amounts of chemical preservatives, served as human guinea pigs to learn about the safety and side effects of food preservatives. Known poisons were prohibited, but the safety of many chemical additives still remained unknown even after their volunteer efforts were over. Passage of the Pesticide Amendment (1954), the Food Additives Amendment (1958), and the Color Additive Amendments (1960) drastically changed the way food manufacturers operated. Up until now, the FDA had regulated foods to ensure safety and wholesomeness and that labeling was truthful and not misleading. Under the Food Additive Amendments the FDA required all new food ingredients to be evaluated for safety, including those used in dietary supplements. For the first time no substance could be introduced into the food supply unless a prior safety determination had been conducted. Food ingredients that were allowed onto the market became known as Generally Recognized As Safe (GRAS) ingredients. According to the FD&C Act:

Under sections 201(s) and 409 of the Federal Food, Drug, and Cosmetic Act (the Act), any substance that is intentionally added to food is a food additive, that is subject to premarket review and approval by FDA, unless the substance is generally recognized, among qualified experts, as having been adequately shown to be safe under the conditions of its intended use, or unless the use of the substance is otherwise excluded from the definition of a food additive. For example, substances whose use meets the definition of a pesticide, a dietary ingredient of a dietary supplement, a color additive, a new animal drug, or a substance approved for such use prior to September 6, 1958, are excluded from the definition of food additive. Sections 201(s) and 409 were enacted in 1958 as part of the Food Additives Amendment to the Act. While it is impracticable to list all ingredients whose use is generally recognized as safe, FDA published a partial list of food ingredients whose use is generally recognized as safe to aid the industry's understanding of what did not require approval.[25]

By 1962, amendments to the FD&C Act were passed, tightening control over prescription, new, and investigational drugs largely because of the thalidomide tragedy in Europe. During the 1950s and 1960s in Europe the drug thalidomide was given to pregnant women for morning sickness. However, safety testing of this drug had been inadequate and resulted in thousands of deformed babies being born. Because of this, drug firms in the United States are now required to send adverse reaction reports to the FDA and list risks and benefits in all advertising. The Good Manufacturing Practice Regulations (GMP) regulations in 1962, which set standards for manufacturing practices used in drug production, were standardized to prevent errors and accidents causing the consumer harm. By 1969 GMPs for food were also established and the FDA, rather than relying on court decisions to enforce laws, now protected consumers through regulations and premarket controls.[26]

Prior to 1994 the FDA maintained tight control over premarket approval of all drugs and foods, including dietary supplements. But in 1976, after years of debate, Congress passed the Proxmire bill that prohibited the FDA from regulating vitamins and minerals as prescription drugs. This eventually led to the passage of DSHEA in 1994, which effectively ended tight FDA control over dietary supplements. The Nutrition Labeling and Education Act of 1990 added "herb, or similar nutritional substances"[27] to the term dietary supplement. With the passage of the Health Freedom Act in 1992, all U.S. citizens were assured the right to choose supposedly safe dietary supplements. By 1994, Congress amended the FD&C Act to include provisions that apply only to dietary supplements and their ingredients. Extensive lobbying efforts by special interest groups and the blanket assumption made by Congress that all supplements were safe led to its eventual passage. Although they recognized the need for more scientific research, the connection between dietary supplement use and disease prevention to reduce spiraling out-of-control health care expenses was appealing. As a result, dietary supplement ingredients no longer undergo premarket safety evaluations and the burden of safety has shifted from the manufacturer to the government and the consumer. Once a dietary supplement is in the market, the FDA must now prove a supplement presents an unreasonable risk of illness or injury to restrict or remove it from the market should problems arise. This change, coupled with chronic understaffing at the FDA, has led to a cumbersome and lengthy process to remove products from the market that pose a potential safety threat. Under DSHEA, a dietary supplement:

- is a product (other than tobacco) that is intended to supplement the diet that bears or contains one or more of the following dietary ingredients: a vitamin,

a mineral, an herb or other botanical, an amino acid, a dietary substance
for use by man to supplement the diet by increasing the total daily intake,
or a concentrate, metabolite, constituent, extract, or combinations of these
ingredients.

- is intended for ingestion in pill, capsule, tablet, or liquid form.
- is not represented for use as a conventional food or as the sole item of a meal
or diet.
- is labeled as a "dietary supplement."
- includes products such as an approved new drug, certified antibiotic, or licensed
biologic that was marketed as a dietary supplement or food before approval,
certification, or license (unless the Secretary of Health and Human Services
waives this provision).[28]

Like almost all foods, dietary supplements must have an ingredient and
nutrient label. Disease claims may not be made about diagnosis, prevention,
treatment or cures, (for example, a product cannot claim to cure cancer or treat
arthritis). But manufacturers can describe supplement effect on "structure or
function" of the body (for example, folic acid can reduce the risk of neural
tube birth defects; vitamin E promotes a healthy heart; or calcium may reduce
the risk of osteoporosis). The manufacturer must be able to substantiate any
statements made to be truthful and not misleading, but FDA approval is not
required.

A second and separate government agency, the Federal Trade Commission
(FTC), is also involved with dietary supplement regulation. The FTC is charged
with truth in advertising—that is, assuring that reliable scientific evidence cor-
roborates truthful advertising statements that are not misleading. Supplement
labels must bear the statement "This statement has not been evaluated by the
Food and Drug Administration. This product is not intended to diagnose, treat,
cure, or prevent any disease." If new ingredients are used the manufacturers
must notify the FDA at least seventy-five days before marketing the product
and provide information about the ingredients that they conclude are safe.
Adverse reactions are reported to the FDA, but reporting is strictly voluntary, unlike the mandatory reporting system that is required for all OTC and
pharmaceutical drugs.[29]

Two government agencies were created to investigate complementary
medicine when DSHEA was enacted and as public health concerns began
to grow. The Office of Dietary Supplements (ODS) was established within the
NIH in the Office of Disease Prevention in 1995 and the National Center for
Complementary and Alternative Medicine (NCCAM), also established within
the NIH, in 1992. The responsibilities of the ODS are to explore the role
dietary supplements play as part of improving health care in the United States
by promoting, conducting, and coordinating scientific research. The ODS also
acts as an advisor to the Secretary and Assistant Secretary for Health, Director of NIH, Director of CDC, and Commissioner of the FDA on all matters
related to dietary supplements.[30] The NCCAM investigates and evaluates un-
conventional medical practices. Their primary focus is to advance scientific

research, train CAM researchers, provide timely and accurate information to health professionals and the public, and support integration of proven CAM therapies.[31]

DSHEA opened a Pandora's box. It appears the intent of DSHEA was to allow more products into the marketplace that might benefit the consumer, but the result has been far different. The authority of the FDA to protect the public has been diminished and it is unable to prevent entry of dietary supplements into the market or quickly act when harm occurs. The result is that dietary supplements in the United States are basically unregulated at this time.

The most publicized and egregious example of ephedra dietary supplements highlights just how much public risk has increased since DSHEA was enacted. Also known as ma huang, ephedra has been used in Chinese medicine for thousands of years for cold and asthma symptoms. The alkaloids ephedrine and pseudoephedrine are the primary active ingredients used in OTC bronchodilators and decongestant medicines (i.e., Claritin) in the United States. They are strictly regulated in these products because they are classified as a drug. But not so when it comes to dietary supplements.

Ephedrine-containing dietary supplements have been advertised in the United States as weight loss aids, energy enhancers, alternatives to psychoactive drugs, and sports enhancers. While adverse events from ephedrine were reported prior to 1994, they increased dramatically after 1994. In 1995 the FDA Food Advisory Committee reported more than 330 adverse events and 12 deaths directly related to ephedrine use. By 1996, the Texas Department of Health—using data from six Texas Poison Center Networks—reported 500 adverse events, including 8 deaths, between 1993 and 1995 from dietary supplement products containing ephedrine. Reported symptoms from ephedra products at the recommended dosages included nervousness, dizziness, tremor, blood pressure changes, headache, gastrointestinal upset, chest pain, myocardial infarction, hepatitis, seizures, and psychosis. At least twenty states had banned or restricted all products containing ephedrine by 1997.

Testimony by the consumer advocacy group Public Citizen to the committee on dietary supplement safety at the National Academy of Sciences in 2001 reported documented cases of harm from ephedra use. Examples of these specific cases included a 37-year-old woman with no medical history but with therapeutic levels of ephedrine and pseudoephedrine in her bloodstream who had suddenly collapsed and died, and a 36-year-old healthy male athlete who suffered an aortic dissection after ephedra use. The U.S. Navy banned all ephedrine-containing dietary supplements after review of documented medical cases illustrated significant adverse events and deaths from ephedrine-containing dietary supplements. An FDA analysis of dietary supplements associated with adverse events between 1993 and 2001 discovered the following:

- 42% (1,398) of a total of 3,308 adverse events associated with dietary supplements involved ephedra alkaloids;

- 59% (81) of a total 137 reported deaths involved ephedra alkaloids;
- 84% (32) of a total 38 reported heart attacks were associated with ephedra alkaloids;
- 63% (62) of a total 98 reports of cardiac arrhythmias were associated with ephedra alkaloids;
- 63% (91) of a total 144 reports of hypertension were associated with ephedra alkaloids;
- 81% (69) of a total 85 reports of stroke were associated with ephedra alkaloids;
- 58% (70) of a total 121 reports of seizure were associated with ephedra alkaloids.

The American Association of Poison Control Centers reported 1,428 adverse events and the FDA received 2,277 reports of adverse reactions between February 1993 and July 2003. It was obvious that ephedra dietary supplements were dangerous.

In 1997 the FDA proposed a rule to regulate ephedra, which included a warning statement on all dietary ephedra product labels. But the U.S. General Accounting Office believed that the FDA did not have sufficient evidence to regulate ephedra and required the FDA to gather more evidence and open the issue to health professionals, the supplement industry, and the public. It would take six years before the FDA could justify protecting the public from ephedra dietary supplements. The death of Steve Bechler, a 23-year-old MLB Baltimore Orioles' pitcher after taking an ephedrine alkaloid dietary supplement, in 2003 sharpened public and regulatory focus onto ephedra dangers. On December 30, 2003, the FDA issued a consumer alert on all supplements containing ephedrine alkaloids and in 2004 the FDA banned the sale of all dietary supplements containing ephedrine alkaloids.[32]

The FDA has been highly criticized for the length of time it took to ban ephedra, but this illustration highlights just how much DSHEA weakened FDA authority over dietary supplement products. Prior to DSHEA, the FDA would have either prevented ephedra entry into the marketplace in the first place or removed it from the market far more quickly after harm was reported.

Increasing concerns about supplement safety, consumer self-prescribing, and adverse events since the implementation of DSHEA resulted in the passage of the Dietary Supplement and Nonprescription Drug Consumer Protection Act in December 2006. This law will now require dietary supplement manufacturers to notify the FDA of any and all reported serious adverse reactions to their products and require a reporting telephone number on all supplement labels. Even so, this new legislation may not be effective enough to protect the public. Since the FDA ban on ephedra in 2004, the supplement company Nutraceutical International Corporation filed a lawsuit to invalidate the FDA ban and claimed the FDA wrongly regulated ephedra as a drug and did not follow the rules set down by DSHEA and the Congress. In 2005 a federal judge considering this lawsuit ruled for the plaintiff, Nutraceutical International Corp., and struck down the FDA ban on ephedra. These supplements are now once again available (a Google search on the Internet returns 1,640,000 hits as of May 27, 2007, when queried on where to buy ephedra dietary supplements) despite the evidence that they represent a significant health risk. Until the FDA can regain the authority it once had, private lawsuits (after death and injury have already occurred) may very well be the consumers' only recourse.

Although vitamin and mineral preparations have not reported adverse events as severe as ephedra, the potential for a similar scenario exists. Dietary supplement contamination is also a concern. ConsumersLab.com, a privately held company with no ties to manufacturers, evaluates health products and provides information to the consumer. A January 2007 report found that 52 percent of multivitamin preparations tested were contaminated with lead, unable to break apart properly, or contained either more, less, or none of the vitamins and minerals they claimed.[33] Until dietary supplements are more tightly controlled, Americans are playing Russian roulette when purchasing and taking any dietary supplement. Consumers beware!

3

ANTIOXIDANTS AND THE REDOX BIOLOGY OF LIFE

According to a November 30, 2006 *Wall Street Journal*[1] article, resveratrol supplements are the current "hot" supplements in America. They have become so popular with Americans that retailers are unable to keep up with consumer demand. A plant phytochemical, flavonoid and stilbene, and antioxidant molecule, media portrayal of resveratrol as a possible antiaging elixir that is life-prolonging has greatly boosted sales of this dietary supplement. The buzz about resveratrol commenced when investigators from Harvard Medical School published a paper in the journal *Nature* in August 2003 about this phytochemical, which is found in red wine and grape skins.[2] The investigators found that resveratrol directly influenced critical genes and prolonged lifespan by 30 to 70 percent in yeast cells, citing unpublished data of preliminary results that the lifespan of fruit flies and earthworms could also be extended. Subsequent studies have demonstrated resveratrol's capability to improve health and survival of mice on a high-calorie diet.[3] While these results look promising, this prolonged lifespan has been achieved only in the lab and only by using very large doses.

This is only just one illustration of how preliminary data about dietary antioxidant health benefits and their purported ability to save us from chronic disease, and quite possibly reverse the aging process, has gained popularity with the public before scientists can unquestionably prove their benefits to humans. We have seen that antioxidant supplement sales are on the rise and functional food/nutraceutical sales are growing by leaps and bounds. However, conflicting scientific data about their benefits and increasing incidences of reported adverse events raise questions about the wisdom of adding them to an already nutritionally adequate diet. Are antioxidants really our answer to increased longevity and reduced chronic diseases? The answer is far more complex than most of us realize and for the remainder of this chapter we will dive into the complex workings of the antioxidant world.

In very simple terms, dietary antioxidants are substances found in the human diet that have the potential to decrease the adverse effects of free radicals within our bodies. The biomolecules in our bodies undergo many reactions every day that require oxygen. Invariably, these oxygen-using reactions produce products that are called free radicals. Free radicals are highly reactive molecules that cause cell damage and are a byproduct of normal cell metabolism that uses oxygen. Free radicals form when molecules split to unpaired electrons, a process known as oxidation. Oxygen is necessary for life-sustaining metabolic processes. These metabolic processes depend upon the chemical reactions of oxidation and reduction (a chemical reaction that adds electrons to the molecule), or more simply put, the transfer of electrons. But oxygen can have a destructive side, as observed when an apple slice turns brown once exposed to air. These free radicals, coupled with oxidizing agents in our environment (such as pollution), can cause damage to our cells (via oxidative stress) over time and factors into the aging and chronic disease process. Antioxidants can "quench," or stop, free radicals before they cause harm, much like soaking apple slices in lemon juice (that contain high levels of ascorbic acid or vitamin C) prevents the oxidative reaction that occurs when food is exposed to air. However, the effectiveness of an antioxidant depends on the free radical involved. It is also necessary to realize that, in some circumstances, an antioxidant can turn into a pro-oxidant that is capable of creating toxic results. A pro-oxidant is an antioxidant gone bad—instead of quenching free radicals, it becomes a radical itself that causes cell damage. So, as we can see, the story of antioxidants and radicals is far more complex than media reports imply.

REDOX BIOLOGY AND LIFE

The use of antioxidant supplements to quench radicals, thus preventing human disease, is often viewed as the only function of antioxidants and free radicals. In fact, antioxidants and radicals permeate much of the biochemistry of life. Scientists discuss this biochemical relationship between antioxidants and radicals using the language of the redox biology research field. Unlike the perception of the average American, those who study redox biology understand that free radicals are not all bad. But not all antioxidants are all good either. Life is a balance between the two. Antioxidants are used in biological systems to regulate the levels of free radicals, permitting them to perform useful biological functions without causing undesirable damage.[4] Inevitably, some damage to critical molecules of the body does occur and thus repair systems are required to maintain cell viability. This concept will be discussed later, but first we need to define the terms oxidation and reduction.

The human body is comprised of many different cell types that are composed of many types of molecules. These molecules consist of elements made up of atoms that are joined by chemical bonds. Atoms, as you most likely remember from basic grade school science, are made up of a nucleus, neutrons, protons, and electrons. These electrons are involved in chemical reactions and bond atoms together to form a molecule. The behavior of an atom is determined by the number of electrons it gains or loses. The basis of understanding chemistry and biochemical reactions within the body relies on understanding the fact that electrons determine much, if not most, of the chemical properties of elements. In chemical reactions electrons are either shared or exchanged between atoms within molecules. Atoms and molecules can absorb or shed energy as electrons move into or from higher energy level orbits around an atoms nucleus. Atoms are stable when their highest energy level orbits contain paired electrons.

Enzymes are elegant molecules (mostly comprised of proteins) that were retained by life during evolution because of their ability to facilitate and control the orderly and efficient transfer of energy between atoms and molecules. When electrons transfer between molecules, energy is also transferred in reactions referred to as "redox reactions." When a molecule loses an electron, it is said to be oxidized. When a molecule receives an electron, it is said to be reduced. Thus gaining, losing, or sharing electrons results in molecular stability. When electrons are shared covalent bonds are formed that require energy to break. For example, breaking the bond between hydrogen atoms requires 104 kcal/mole of energy from some source. Nearly all of biochemistry involves the transfer of energy by movement of electrons in the formation or breaking of bonds between hydrogen, oxygen, nitrogen, carbon, and sulfur atoms. It can thus be realized that most of the reactions of life involve formation of atoms or groups of atoms capable of independent existence with at least one unpaired electron. Such atoms are known as "radicals." The first ever radical described in organic chemistry, the triphenylmethyl radical, was identified by Moses Gomberg in 1900 while working in Munich.[5]

In 1957, Denham Harman proposed the "free radical theory of aging."[6] His hypothesis suggested that consequences of aging result from attacks by radicals generated primarily in the cell mitochondria during normal metabolism. Because of their unstable nature, highly reactive radicals enter into uncontrolled reactions that damage healthy cell tissue. As the damage to proteins, lipids, and nucleic acids in the body accumulates, aging effects ensue. Harman's theory was controversial at the time[7] since most scientists thought that fleeting radicals were not likely to have a significant impact on the biochemistry of life. Over half a century of research would prove this notion to be naive. The first-hard evidence that free radicals could play a significant role in biology came in 1968 with the discovery of a specific enzyme, superoxide dismutases (SOD), whose function was the detoxification of the superoxide radical.[8] Superoxide is a highly reactive oxygen radical formed by a single electron reduction reaction that occurs during normal cell metabolism. If it is not controlled, devastating cell damage can result. The importance of the SOD enzymes in preventing this damage is demonstrated by the fact that when the manganese SOD gene is "knocked out" or removed in experiments with mice, death will result within ten days after birth.[9]

Once it was established that free radicals could exist and interact with biomolecules, and that there were enzyme systems whose primary function was the "control" of radicals, Harman's theory began to gain acceptance. This concept of radical control carried with it the understanding that radicals were dangerous entities in a biological setting. It was quickly realized that free radicals could easily react with cellular substrates (or biomolecules) such as lipids, proteins, and DNA. When radical production exceeds the ability of an organism to control, prevent, or repair damage from these radicals, a condition termed "oxidative stress" arises. Damage to biomolecules from oxidation disturbs normal cell function. Since radicals are so potentially harmful to biomolecules, many scientists have hypothesized that where the existence of uncontrolled radicals has been observed, diseases are caused by reactive radical species damage and "oxidative stress."

As we saw, many free radicals come into existence as a byproduct of natural cell processes, such as oxygen metabolism or inflammation. For example, when cells use oxygen to oxidize glucose in the mitochondria to generate adenosine triphosphate (ATP) for cellular energy, free radicals are created. Various endogenous oxidases (enzymes that react with oxygen to change a biochemical substrate) can also create radicals as byproducts of their function. Examples of the very basic radical generation and sequestration reactions in biological systems are depicted in Figure 3.1.

Many internal processes, influenced by lifestyle choices, can affect radical levels. Cigarette smoking and excessive consumption of alcohol result in measurably increased levels of radicals. Exogenous sources and environmental conditions can create radicals from ionizing radiation (sun exposure, cosmic rays, medical X-rays, or industrial processes), environmental toxins, and atmospheric pollution (ozone or nitric oxide produced from motor exhaust) as well. Biological systems have evolved to control or sequester these radicals and still other systems have evolved to repair cell damage once it occurs. But before we can explore them further, some additional definitions are necessary.

DEFINING FREE RADICALS, ANTIOXIDANTS, AND RELATED TERMS

The terms "reactive oxygen species" (ROS) and "reactive nitrogen species" (RNS) describe both radicals and nonradical reactive oxygen and nitrogen-containing molecules. These molecules can enter reactions that can result in production of free radicals or directly damage organic biochemical substrates. The nomenclature used within the field of free radical biology has not been established by any one organization. However, there is a consensus within the field from several sources, including the International Union of Pure and Applied Chemistry (IUPAC),[10] the Commission on the Nomenclature of Inorganic Chemistry,[11] and by recommendations of authors in the field.[12] Current convention denotes a free radical in text by a superscript dot to the right preceding any charge that the molecule may have, for example $H^{\bullet}$, $HO^{\bullet}$, $NO^{\bullet}$, $O_2^{\bullet -}$, $CO_2^{\bullet -}$, and $H_3C^{\bullet}$. $O_2^{2\bullet}$ denotes the radical notation for dioxygen in its ground state or, in other words, the lowest allowed energy state for this molecule. A molecule is capable of being highly reactive even if it

Figure 3.1
Basic Radical Generation and Sequestration Reactions

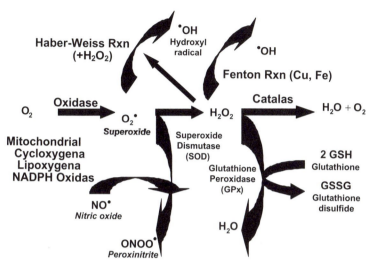

Oxygen enters the biological system and is used in the mitochondria in the creation of ATP. It is also used by various other oxidase enzymes in the cell during normal metabolism. A byproduct of these processes is the superoxide radical that must be dealt with by superoxide dismutase and catalase to convert it to harmless water and oxygen before it does damage. If superoxide reacts with either nitric oxide (another radical) or hydrogen peroxide peroxynitrite, the hydroxyl radicals are produced (two very reactive and dangerous radicals). When superoxide dismutase converts superoxide to hydrogen peroxide in biological systems, there are four possible fates for the hydrogen peroxide. If either the catalase or the glutathione peroxidase enzymes deal with it, hydrogen peroxide is converted safely to harmless products. However, when hydrogen peroxide enters either a Haber-Weiss reaction with superoxide or the Fenton reaction, which unsequesters metals, dangerous hydroxyl radicals can be produced that can cause biological damage.

is not technically a radical (if its electrons are paired). Common biologically relevant oxygen and nitrogen radicals are listed in Table 3.1, together with other highly reactive nonradical biologically important oxygen and nitrogen molecules.

Beyond the simple small molecular weight radicals, biological reactions can produce many other radicals from biomolecules. For example, phenolic and other aromatic radical molecules as well as superoxide radicals are often formed during xenobiotic metabolism as part of natural detoxification mechanisms depicted in Figure 3.2. The term xenobiotic was coined to cover all organic compounds that were foreign to the organism under study. Pesticides are a common example of a xenobiotic compound.

Table 3.1
Common Biological Radical and Non-Radical Species

Reactive Oxygen Species (ROS)		
Common Name	Radical Depiction	Systemic Name
	Radicals	
Radical anion of $HO^\bullet$	$O^{\bullet-}$	oxide($\bullet 1-$)
Superoxide	$O_2^{\bullet-}$	dioxide($\bullet 1-$)
	$O_2^{\bullet+}$	dioxygen($\bullet 1+$)
oxygen, written as O_2	$O_2^{2\bullet}$	dioxygen (triplet)
ozonide	$O_3^{\bullet-}$	trioxide($\bullet 1-$)
hydroxyl	$HO^\bullet$	hydridooxygen
Hydroperoxyl	$HO_2^\bullet$	hydridodioxygen($\bullet$)
hydrogen trioxide radical	HO_3	hydridotrioxygen($\bullet$)
carbon dioxide radical anion	$CO_2^{\bullet-}$	dioxidocarbonate ($\bullet 1-$)
carbonate radical	$CO_3^{\bullet-}$	trioxidocarbonate($\bullet 1-$)
	$HOCO^\bullet$	hydroxidooxidocarbon($\bullet$)
	$HOCO_2^\bullet$	hydroxidodioxidocarbon($\bullet$)
Peroxyl Radical	$RO_2^\bullet$	
Alkoxyl Radical Water	$RO^\bullet$	
	Nonradicals	
Water	H_2O	
Hydrogen Peroxide	H_2O_2	
Ozone	O_3	
Singlet Oxygen	$1\Delta g$	

Reactive Nitrogen Species (RNS)		
	Radicals	
Nitric Oxide	$NO^\bullet$	oxidonitrogen ($\bullet$)
nitroxyl	$NO_{(2}^\bullet)^-$	oxidonitrate($2\bullet 1-$) (triplet)
Nitrogen dioxide	NO_2	dioxidonitrogen
nitrogen trioxide	$NO_3^\bullet$	trioxidonitrogen($\bullet$)
	$NO_2^{\bullet 2-}$	dioxidonitrate($\bullet 2-$)
	$NO_3^{\bullet 2-}$	trioxidonitrate($\bullet 2-$)
peroxynitrite	$ONOO^\bullet$	(dioxido)oxidonitrogen($\bullet$)
	$HON_2^\bullet$	hydroxidonitrogen($2\bullet$) (triplet)
	$(NO)_2^{\bullet-}$	bis(oxidonitrate)(N − N)($\bullet 1-$)
	$N_2O^{\bullet-}$	oxidodinitrate($\bullet 1-$)
azidyl radical	$N_3^\bullet$	trinitrogen(2N − N)($\bullet$)
	Nonradicals	
Nitrous acid	$HNO2$	
Dinitrogen tetroxide	$N2O4$	
Dinitrogen trioxide	$N2O3$	
Peroxynitrite	$ONOO^-$	
Peroxynitrous acid	$ONOOH$	
Nitonium cation	NO_2^+	
Alkyl peroxynitrites	$ROONO$	

Table 3.1 *(continued)*

Common Name	Radical Depiction	Systemic Name
	Other Reactive Species	
hypochlorite	OCl⁻	oxidochlorate(1−)
hypochlorous acid	HOCl	hydrogenoxidochlorate
hypobromite	OBr⁻	oxidobromate(1−)
hypobromous acid	HOBr	hydrogenoxidobromate
hypoiodite	OI⁻	oxidoiodate(1−)
hypoiodous acid	HOI	hydrogenoxidoiodate
hypothiocyanate	OSCN−	oxidothiocyanate(1−)
hypothiocyanous acid	HOSCN	hydrogenoxidothiocyanate

Figure 3.2
Xenobiotic Metabolism

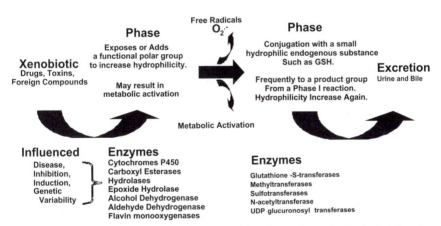

When a foreign molecule that has the potential to be toxic to the body is taken in, xenobiotic metabolism modifies the molecule using a variety of enzymes that expose or add polar groups to it and mark it for removal. Making a molecule more polar makes it more hydrophilic and thus easier to remove from the body. This process sometimes produces free radicals or radicals of the xenobiotic, both of which can cause potential damage. Such "activated molecules have also been implicated in cancer etiology. In a second phase of detoxification other enzymes add thiol, methyl, sulfur, acetyl, or glucuronyl groups to detoxify Phase 1 metabolites and render them even more hydrophilic for removal. The endogenous antioxidant glutathione is important to both radical quenching after Phase 1 and to Phase 2 enzymatic processes.

Radical molecules may also combine together or with other reactive molecules generating yet more damaging radicals. An example is the reaction between superoxide and nitric oxide that produces peroxynitrite (ONOO$^{\bullet}$), a highly reactive and dangerous radical. Under certain conditions of hypoxia (decreased oxygen to cell tissues that can occur, for instance, in anemia or stroke), the enzyme xanthine oxidase can simultaneously create both these radicals in close proximity in tissues and thus intensify damage done to biological tissues.[13]

Not all ROS and RNS are true radicals because some have paired electrons. To be a radical, a molecule must have unpaired electrons. The most common ROS and RNS (radical and otherwise) are listed in Table 3.1. Numerous *in vitro* studies have shown that ROS and RNS can easily react with many other biomolecules, causing dysfunction of the integral components of the cell. In fact, much experimental data exists to indicate that lipid peroxidation, protein oxidation, and oxidative alterations to nucleic acids mediated by ROS and RNS are crucial components of the damaging actions of these compounds. Many studies show that dietary antioxidants, which include vitamin C (ascorbic acid), vitamin E (α-tocopherol), β-carotene (a carotenoid), and flavonoids (a subgroup of the phytochemicals), when used within experimental *in vitro* biological systems, act as effective antioxidants protecting plasma components, including lipoproteins, and cells from damage.[14]

So what exactly are antioxidants? Chemists define an antioxidant as "any substance that, when present in low concentrations compared to that of an oxidizable substrate, significantly delays or inhibits the oxidation of that substrate."[15] Thoughtful consideration of this definition leads to the inevitable conclusion that an enormous number of biological compounds can act as antioxidants. All compounds or molecules can be ranked on the basis of their "oxidation potential." This ranking is based on the electrochemical potential at which the transfer of an electron will occur and the compound will be oxidized. As a general rule, any molecule with a higher oxidation potential in comparison to a lower oxidation potential molecule can oxidize that molecule. Lipid peroxidation (damage to polyunsaturated fatty acids [PUFA]) usually occurs by an initial reaction with highly reactive radicals. In this case, let's consider the hydroxyl radical that has an oxidation potential at pH 7.0 of 2310 mV, a physical measure of the energy required to remove yet another electron for this molecule. In order for the hydroxyl radical to stabilize itself, it needs to take an electron from any molecule that has an oxidation potential lower than 2310 mV. The lower the oxidation potential of the other molecule, the more easily the hydroxyl radical can take an electron. The hydrogen atom from the bis-allylic position on PUFAs (the double bonds PUFAs can have in their molecular structure which make them more susceptible to free radical attacks and oxidation) oxidizes at 600 mV. This is much lower than that of the hydroxyl radical's oxidation potential. This means that the reaction between the PUFA and the hydroxyl radical will occur easily, stabilizing the hydroxyl radical by acquiring an electron and "reducing" the hydroxyl radical to water so it is no longer harmful. But damage has already been done to the PUFA, turning it into a pentadienyl radical (PUFA$^\bullet$). The PUFA$^\bullet$ radical can now react with oxygen to form a new unstable radical called peroxyl radical within the PUFA molecule (ROO$^\bullet$). This new peroxyl radical reacts easily with other PUFA molecules and damage to lipids continues in a chain reaction progression much like a fire out of control damaging many other PUFA molecules in the process. This chain reaction process is driven by the continued production of new peroxyl radicals as long as there is lipid to oxidize, or until another molecule with a lower oxidation potential than PUFA is introduced into the system. Vitamin E (α-tocopherol) has an oxidation potential of 500 mV (100 mV lower than that of PUFA's) and can also react with the peroxyl radical, thus reducing it and preventing it from producing more radicals in the chain reaction. Vitamin E can also react with hydroxyl radicals that initially start the chain reaction and thus can prevent the first steps in oxidizing PUFAs. Therefore, vitamin E is both a preventive and a chain-breaking antioxidant. But there is one caveat: when vitamin E is oxidized it yields its electron regardless of the radical it reduced. The α-tocopherol molecule left has an unpaired electron and now becomes a radical itself. Fortunately, in biological systems, the α-tocopherol radical is a relatively stable radical. However, in its radical form it is no longer capable of protecting lipids from oxidation by other radicals. Vitamin C (ascorbate) has an oxidation potential of 282 mV and is capable of reacting with the α-tocopherol radical and thereby restoring the original "reduced" vitamin E and effectively "recycling" vitamin E. By now you should know what comes next. Vitamin C, by reducing vitamin E, now becomes a radical known as the ascorbate radical. If this appears to be a "pecking order," that's because it is. In the rank order of biological molecules based on their oxidation potential, each molecule higher on the list can potentially oxidize any molecule lower on the list. An example of this is shown in Table 3.2. Although this concept has always been intuitive to redox chemists, it has only been taught to students and scientists in free radical biology and biochemistry since its introduction by G.R. Buettner in 1993.[16]

Among the low-molecular-weight antioxidants in biological systems, vitamin C (ascorbate) appears to be a necessary component for the life functions of both higher plants and animals. Many animals possess the ability to synthesize vitamin C, but humans do not. Thus, in humans, vitamin C is an essential nutrient. The same holds true for vitamin E. Vitamin C's presence at what is considered a high physiological concentration in the millimolar range in many if not all cells of the body hints at its critical nature. Surprisingly, although it has been long known that vitamin C was present in plants since 1933, only recently has progress been made in understanding the biosynthetic pathways.[17]

Another important small molecular weight antioxidant in plants, animals, and humans is the molecule glutathione (GSH). This ever-present tripeptide L-glutathione (GSH or gamma-glutamyl-cysteinyl-glycine) is a well-known biological antioxidant and theorized to be the primary intracellular antioxidant for higher organisms. When oxidized, it forms oxidized glutathione (GSSG), which

Table 3.2
The Pecking Order Based on Oxidation Potential

Redox Couple One Electron Reductions	$E^{\circ\prime}/mV$
$HO^{\bullet}$, H^{+}/H_2O	+2310
$RO^{\bullet}$, H^{+}/ROH (aliphatic alkoxyl radical)	+1600
$ROO^{\bullet}$, $H^{+}/ROOH$ (alkyl peroxyl radical)	+1000
$GS^{\bullet}/GS^{-}$ (glutathione)	+920
$PUFA^{\bullet}$, $H^{-}/PUFA\text{-}H$ (bis-alkylic-H)	+600
$TO^{\bullet}$, H^{+}/TOH (vitamin E)	+480
H_2O_2, H^{+}/H_2O, $HO^{\bullet}$	+320
$Asc^{\bullet-}$, $H^{+}/AscH^{-}$ (vitamin C)	+282
Coenzyme $Q^{\bullet-}$, $2H^{+}/$Coenzyme QH_2	+200
Iron (III) EDTA/ Iron (II) EDTA	+120
Coenzyme $Q/$Coenzyme $Q^{\bullet-}$	−36
$O_2 / O_2^{\bullet-}$	−160
$RSSR / RSSR^{\bullet-}$ (GSH)	−1500
H_2O/ e^{-}_{aq}	−2870

Note: The hydroxyl radical is reduced by the PUFA or the vitamin E below it in the table. In turn, the resulting vitamin E radical is reduced by ascorbate below it in the table and in turn the ascorbate radical is reduced by reduced glutathione (GSH). Adapted from Buettner (1993).[18]

is easily recycled in any living cell that produces the enzyme glutathione reductase. GSH passes easily through cell membranes[19] and GSH functions directly or indirectly in many important biological enzymatic and metabolic processes, including the synthesis of proteins and DNA, as well as protecting cells from free-radical mediated damage. GSH is critical in cellular maintenance of a proper oxidation state within the body.[20] GSH is synthesized by most cells and also supplied in the diet.

Approximately 7–8 grams of reduced GSH produced in the human body daily is generated from GSSG primarily by the liver, and to a smaller extent, by the skeletal muscle and blood cells. The remaining 1 or 2 grams found in the body is acquired from dietary sources. A deficiency of GSH in cells can quickly lead to excess free radicals in the cell that can lead to oxidative stress. However, inadequate levels of GSH can also lead to the accumulation of toxins as a result of inadequate Phase 2 metabolism. These two consequences will ultimately lead to cell death. With an oxidation potential of 80 mV, GSH can reduce most of the dangerous radicals produced in biological systems as well as recycle both vitamin E and vitamin C.

Case-controlled studies have adequately demonstrated that biomarkers of oxidative damage in humans increase with age. Age-related disorders and diseases, such as Alzheimer's, neurodegenerative diseases, cancer, autoimmune diseases, rheumatoid arthritis, diabetes, and cardiovascular disease, with radical involvement are hypothesized to be the end result.[21]

Despite clear evidence of increased oxidative damage with age and age-related diseases, it still has not been proven *in vivo* that pretreatment with antioxidants will prevent tissue damage. To make matters worse, some studies have even produced data that antioxidant treatment not only failed to restore pathologies where ROS were purported to play a causal role, but appeared to even make injury worse.[22] Furthermore, molecular studies are demonstrating crucial roles for ROS in signaling mechanisms both within and between cells that are necessary to maintain normal function.[23] As a result, a number of scientists have come to the conclusion that the excessive production of ROS is actually the consequence, rather than the root cause, of health disorders and diseases.[24] Concepts currently evolving in the field of radical biology and medicine theorize that free radicals have become vital in the functioning of every air-living organism because of the way life evolved on earth. However, if systems that have evolved to control radicals are compromised or become dysfunctional, uncontrolled radicals can cause damage to critical biomolecules necessary for life. If this damage is not repaired, organ function can eventually be impaired leading inevitably to disease, aging, and death.

EVOLUTION OF LIFE AND THE ROLE OF OXYGEN

Evolution has produced a fascinating paradox that exists in the biochemistry of all existing aerobic organisms. The emergence of photosynthesis 3.5 billion years ago, along with cyanobacterial dominance over the preceding billion years, fundamentally changed the earth's atmosphere from a reducing environment to an oxidizing environment via the introduction of atmospheric oxygen.

Photosynthesis is the process by which plants as well as some bacteria and some protistans (one cell organisms) use the energy from sunlight to produce glucose from carbon dioxide and water. Photosynthesis may be summarized by the word equation:

$$\text{carbon dioxide} + \text{water} \xrightarrow[\text{chlorophyll}]{\text{sunlight}} \text{glucose} + \text{oxygen}$$

Beginning in the middle proterozoic period, some 2 billion years ago, oxygen build-up in the atmosphere led to widespread bacterial extinction. But this also produced the evolution of antioxidant defensive biochemical pathways in surviving bacterial and eukaryotic life forms, including multicellular algae.[25] Today, the bulk of animals on earth need O_2 for efficient production of energy in cell mitochondria. This need for O_2 obscures the fact that oxygen is actually a toxic gas. Existing anaerobe bacteria that survived the proterozoic extinction event by "hiding" in anaerobic environments die in the presence of O_2 today. It is also true that all aerobes living today survive because their predecessors evolved antioxidant defenses.[26] The dominance of cyanobacteria for billions of years was grounded in their ability to use the sun's energy to split water. Thus, reducing power (hydrogen equivalents) was attained to drive their metabolism. The byproduct, large amounts of O_2, was discarded into the atmosphere as air pollution. Initially, most of this O_2 was consumed in the formation of metallic oxide deposits that can be seen in rock and ore deposits today, and are most evident as the red oxides of iron in geologic strata. Only when these deposits were saturated did O_2 begin to build up in the atmosphere. The rise in atmospheric O_2 was advantageous to life on earth in at least two ways. First, it led to the formation of the ozone (O_3) layer in the stratosphere that protects living organisms from UV-C radiation. This factor may have been critical in the emergence of organisms from the sea and their ability to colonize land. The rise of atmospheric oxygen also removed ferrous iron (Fe^{2+}) from aqueous environments by forming insoluble ferric complexes. Most of the earths crust (Fe^{2+}) was precipitated from solution, leaving sea and river waters today containing only trace amounts of soluble iron.[27] What was the advantage of removing Fe^{2+}? This species (Fe^{2+}) reacts rapidly with hydrogen peroxide (H_2O_2) to yield highly toxic hydroxyl radicals in the following reactions:

$$Fe^{2+} + H_2O_2 \rightarrow Fe^{3+} + HO^{\bullet} + OH^-$$
$$Fe^{3+} + H_2O_2 \rightarrow Fe^{2+} + HOO^{\bullet} + H^+$$

This reaction, called the Fenton reaction, has been recognized since 1876. Fenton chemistry occurs *in vivo*, but organisms carefully control it by binding Fe^{2+} to carrier proteins and enzymatic reactions that limit concentrations of H_2O_2. It is unlikely that aerobic life could have easily evolved if free Fe^{2+} remained common in the environment. When living organisms first appeared on Earth, they did so under an atmosphere containing much N_2 and CO_2, but little O_2 (i.e., they were anaerobes).[28] As mentioned, anaerobes still exist today, but usually their growth is inhibited or they perish by exposure to the current atmospheric level of 21 percent O_2. As a result, they exist in largely anoxic microenvironments. To exploit environmental niches high in oxygen, other organisms began to evolve antioxidant defenses to protect against O_2 toxicity by producing new molecules expressly for this purpose. These molecules were, however, simply retooled ancient molecules applied to new functions. It has been suggested that the earliest of these molecules were proteins capable of binding to and detoxifying iron, thereby protecting DNA against the Fenton chemistry of the period.[29] In retrospect, this development of antioxidants was a fruitful path for life forms to follow. Organisms that tolerated O_2 could further evolve to use it for metabolic transformations catalyzed by new oxidase, oxygenase, and hydroxylase enzymes (such as lysine and proline hydroxylases) necessary for the biosynthesis of collagen. Indeed, large multicellular animals, evolving by the late proterozoic period, require collagen as an important component of support tissues (bone and cartilage). Perhaps more important than any of these developments was the creation of new and efficient energy production pathways that employed electron-transport chains and utilized O_2 as the terminal electron acceptor. Rapid evolution followed, made possible by the sudden (evolutionarily speaking) availability of cellular energy that was in excess of fundamental life needs. This progression was set in motion by the occurrence of a symbiotic relationship that led to the development of eukaryote cells—cells with mitochondria and the capability of conducting oxidative phosphorylation (cellular respiration).

This switch to aerobic metabolism, using oxidative phosphorylation, increased the yield of ATP that could be made from food molecules, such as glucose, over fifteen-fold. The existence of a new and efficient energy production system allowed the evolution of complex multicellular organisms, which then required systems to ensure that O_2 could be distributed throughout their bodies.[30] The advantage to evolving systems that delivered O_2 throughout the body was that the level of tissue O_2 could be controlled. For example, oxygen is delivered by blood via the circulatory system and partial pressure of O_2 in blood is limited to a level between $10-12$ percent O_2, much lower than that of air. Another step down in O_2 concentration occurs as O_2 is transferred to tissues where levels become only $3-6$ percent of atmospheric levels.[31] As a result, cells in tissue are never exposed to the full force of atmospheric O_2.

Thus we arrive at the great biochemical paradox in the biochemistry of aerobic organisms. Evolution presents life forms with a complex series of tradeoffs, providing organisms with survival advantages and disadvantages. To gain increased production of cellular energy (ATP) by mitochondria via oxidative phosphorylation, and a resulting survival advantage in their *in situ* environment, organisms developed a system to manage high energy biological packets. Those systems, however, are capable of producing toxic reactive species capable of modifying or damaging other critical cellular molecules.[32] In another interesting twist of later evolution, organisms also began to utilize radicals as cellular secondary messengers and in redox signaling mechanisms. Animals have even evolved strategies to incorporate ROS as biological weapons in defense mechanisms that kill bacteria such as that accomplished via the macrophage respiratory burst.[33] Thus, we see the paradoxical result that animals cannot live without oxygen, yet oxygen will ultimately lead to their eventual demise.

One puzzling question has confounded scientist for decades—how could photosynthetic organisms producing poisonous O_2 have evolved? This question was simply stated by Barry Halliwell who asked, "How could cyanobacteria evolve photosynthesis in a pre-antioxidant world?"[34] The gravity of the problem can be seen in the fact that even in present-day plants, which are full of antioxidants, much of the protein synthetic activity of chloroplasts is used to replace photo-oxidatively damaged proteins in the photosynthetic machinery of the chloroplast. Were antioxidants present in early cells and were they at levels sufficiently high to permit evolutionary "experimentation" with photosynthesis? Speculation suggests that the current photosystem PSII existing in today's plants evolved from a manganese-containing form of the enzyme catalase.[35] These enzymes catalyze the rapid breakdown of H_2O_2 in both plants and animals.[36] While most catalases are heme-containing proteins (red pigments containing iron to which O_2 binds), bacteria exist today that still contain catalases with manganese at their active sites.[37] Catalases facilitate the illustrated equation below:

$$\text{Catalase}$$
$$2H_2O_2 \quad \rightarrow \quad O_2 + 2H_2O$$

If the hypothesis that manganese catalases evolved into components of the present day plant photosystem PSII are true, then catalase-like enzymes might have been present in bacteria prior to a rise in atmospheric O_2. Was the presence of H_2O_2 a driving reason for the evolution of these "endogenous" bacterial oxidative defense enzymes? Earths' early atmosphere was composed of N_2 and CO_2 with very little ozone (O_3) to act as a UV screen. Thus, UV radiation at the earth's surface must have been intense. Consequently, the low O_2 levels (as low as 0.1 percent) existing 3.5 billion years ago could have supported photochemical generation of substantial amounts of H_2O_2. Fe^{2+} existed at very high levels at the time and whatever H_2O_2 that was formed would react quickly with it. As a consequence, Fenton chemistry would have been a deadly threat to life. Clearly, H_2O_2 had to be eliminated before Fenton chemistry resulted in generation of highly dangerous hydroxyl radicals that could lead to serious biological damage. Catalases did this job for early life forms and they still eliminate H_2O_2 for higher organisms today.

It has been proposed that during evolution, early photosynthetic systems used H_2O_2 as a substrate[38] and the ability to split the bonds of water was developed later in the evolution of current-day photosynthesis. There is evidence that atmospheric O_2 levels on Earth were higher at one point than current levels. Plant life was exceedingly abundant during the Carboniferous era, 360 million years to 286 million years ago, and this abundance not only isolated CO_2 into large coal and oil deposits, but also increased atmospheric O_2 levels to as much as 35 percent.[39] Evidence of higher oxygen levels is seen in the geologic record of the existence of giant insects during the late Paleozoic era, 543 to 248 million years ago.[40] Such insects could not have existed without higher atmospheric levels of oxygen because of the way insects deliver oxygen to their tissues. Likewise their mass extinction, which occurred during the subsequent Permian-Triassic transition some 250 million years ago, may have been due to more hypoxic atmospheric conditions.[41] Regardless of whether atmospheric oxygen levels regulate the size of our largest insects, all life needs to maintain tissue levels of O_2 within relatively small safety margins or risk high levels of radical induced damage. Plants and animals of the Carboniferous era may have exhibited enhanced antioxidant defenses, but we will never completely know. It is an intriguing fact, however, that evolutionary ancient plant species that evolved during the Carboniferous era, and still exist substantially unchanged today, are better equipped to utilize O_2 as an electron acceptor and to resist oxidative damage than more recently evolved plants.[42] Many of these enzyme-based defense systems are highly conserved throughout evolution and the most important classes are represented by the enzymes listed in Table 3.3, the actions of which will be discussed later. For many of these enzymes, several forms exist in tissues of the body and when combined, represent the first line of defense against oxidative damage.

Table 3.3
Important Antioxidant Enzymes

Common Name	Abbreviation in Text	EC Enzyme Number
Superoxide Dismutase	SOD1 is located in the cytoplasm CuZnSOD SOD2 in the mitochondria MnSOD SOD3 is extracellular. EC(CuZn)SOD and ECMnSOD	EC 1.15.1.1
Catalases	CAT	EC 1.11.1.6
NADH peroxidase		EC 1.11.1.1
NADPH peroxidase		EC 1.11.1.2
fatty-acid peroxidase		EC 1.13.11.11
cytochrome-c peroxidase		EC 1.11.1.5
peroxidase		EC 1.11.1.7
iodide peroxidase		EC 1.11.1.8
chloride peroxidase		EC 1.11.1.10
manganese peroxidase		EC 1.11.1.13
lignin peroxidase		EC 1.11.1.14
versatile peroxidase		EC 1.11.1.16
phospholipid-hydroperoxide glutathione peroxidase	PH-GPx	EC 1.11.1.12
glutathione peroxidase	GPx	EC 1.11.1.9
glutathione reductases	GR	EC 1.8.1.7
glutathione transferase	GST	EC 2.5.1.18
peroxiredoxin (thioredoxin peroxidases)	TRx	EC 1.11.1.15
thioredoxin-disulfide reductase	TRxR or TR	EC 1.8.1.9
L-ascorbate peroxidase	APx	EC 1.11.1.11
monodehydroascorbate reductase (NADH)	MDHAR	EC 1.6.5.4
quinone reductases (NADPH)	QR	EC 1.6.5.5

OXYGEN TOXICITY

All aerobic life forms, from bacteria to humans, suffer damage when exposed to elevated O_2 concentrations. This damage is believed to be due to the formation of the superoxide radical $(O_2^{\bullet -})$.[43] The O_2 molecule is a free radical because there are two unpaired electrons in its outermost orbit that have the same spin quantum number (or parallel spins). While this represents a radical state for O_2, it is nevertheless at its most stable state and exists as such in the atmosphere. In chemical terms, O_2 is an oxidizing and potent agent. If this is so, what keeps it from immediately oxidizing every molecule it comes in contact with? The answer is found in the two unpaired electrons that exist in parallel spins. In order for O_2 to take a pair of electrons from (oxidize) another molecule, both captured electrons must also have parallel spins. Since most stable molecules have paired electrons spinning in opposite directions, O_2 reacts slowly or not at all. O_2 does, however, react actively with other radicals where it takes single electrons immediately.

Biological materials are oxidized by O_2 during combustion because they are heated to the extent that chemical bonds are broken and radicals are formed. O_2 reacts with these radicals and more bonds can be broken with the aid of the additional heat released and available to the system. Thus, lacking the conditions of combustion, ground state O_2 reacts sluggishly with organic molecules. There are, however, other forms of O_2 that are more reactive. Energy from sources such as radiation can be sufficient to rearrange O_2 electrons, thus eliminating the spin restriction to radical reaction and forming what is called a singlet oxygen.[44] When energy from photosynthesis is not handled properly, chlorophyll can transfer energy onto ground-state O_2 producing singlet oxygen.[45] Plants have evolved to utilize molecules called carotenoids to quench both singlet oxygen and the triplet state chlorophyll molecules that can produce it. β-carotene is one example of these carotenoids. Singlet oxygen can also be formed in animal tissues, such as the eye and skin, exposed to solar or other radiation. However, the most common active form of O_2 arises from the addition of a single electron to it forming the superoxide radical $(O_2^{\bullet -})$. Addition of yet another electron leads to generation of the peroxide ion. Addition of more electrons will break bonds and with subsequent reduction reactions (using two or four hydrogen atoms), these dangerous species are changed to H_2O_2 or water.

In eukaryotic cells this reduction of O_2 to water is accomplished by the mitochondria as they break apart glucose in the production of ATP for cell use as energy. Using the cytochrome oxidase multiprotein assembly complex, the mitochondria reduce more than 95 percent of utilized O_2 to water. While the cytochrome complex is efficient in controlling these dangerous partially reduced oxygen species as they are reduced to water, the mitochondrial electron transport chain is not perfect.[46] Indeed, mitochondria are the highest endogenous source of radicals in the cell. Imperfect mitochondrial electron transport results in one-electron reduction of O_2 to form $O_2^{\bullet -}$ and the spontaneous and enzymatic dismutation of $O_2^{\bullet-}$ yields H_2O_2. Consequently, significant byproducts of a flawed sequence of oxidation-reduction reactions in the mitochondia produce radicals that sometimes escape to either be quenched by antioxidants or to cause biological damage. This has lead to several theories of aging based on metabolic rate, mitochondrial damage, or damage to the mitochondria's own DNA by its own production of radicals.

ANTIOXIDANT DEFENSES

As discussed, the most significant sources of oxygen radicals in aerobic plant and animal cells come from the electron-transport chains of the chloroplasts (in plants) and mitochondria (in both plants and animals). Uncoupling proteins exist in the inner mitochondrial membranes of plants and animals that have been proposed as initial antioxidants, acting as an engine vent and permitting increased proton leakage into the mitochondria. This in turn minimizes the accumulation of excessive electrons in the chain that could escape to O_2 and result in oxygen radical formation.[47]

If superoxide is produced within cell tissues, the superoxide dismutase enzymes (SODs) remove it by "dismutation," a process where two radicals are eliminated by reduction of one to H_2O_2 and oxidation of the other to O_2. There are two SODs present in animal tissues. One is exclusively a mitochondrial matrix enzyme and employs manganese within its active-site (MnSOD). Another contains copper and zinc in its active site (CuZnSOD) and exists in the mitochondrial and the cytosol of animal cells.[48] The process of removing superoxide requires the actions of both superoxide dismutases and reductases as well as the catalases necessary to remove H_2O_2, one of the products of these enzyme reactions. Another important class of enzymes capable of removing H_2O_2 is the glutathione peroxidases.[49] Glutathione peroxidases (GPx) require selenium as a cofactor in their activity, which involves removing H_2O_2 by reducing it to water while oxidizing the tripeptide (glu-cys-gly) known as GSH. This activity is explained by the equation:

$$\text{glutathione peroxidases}$$
$$H_2O_2 + 2GSH \quad \rightarrow \quad 2H_2O + GSSG$$

The product of the action of GPx, oxidized glutathione (GSSG), can be converted back to GSH by glutathione reductase enzymes. There are four types of GPx in animal tissues and they all require selenium for activity. This has led to the misconception that selenium is an antioxidant. Selenium, in reality, is a cofactor. Because of this incorporation of selenium, GPx are referred to as selenoproteins. Plant GPx are not dependant upon selenium, but they are less potent than their animal selenoprotein counterparts. In addition, plant GPx tend to utilize thioredoxin (proteins that act as antioxidants) rather than GSH as their hydrogen donors in their reduction reactions. This observation led researchers to the discovery that animal cells also contain thioredoxin-utilizing peroxidases that amount to as much as 0.8 percent of total soluble protein in some cells.[50] This propensity, from bacterial forms to higher plants and animals, to utilize thiols (sulfur and hydrogen atoms) in reduction reactions to remove dangerous reactive oxygen species has its basis in the origin of life in a thiol-rich reducing environment. When thioredoxins are oxidized by H_2O_2, they can be recycled by the reduction reaction thioredoxin reductase, another selenoprotein. The requirement for selenium in the glutathione peroxidases and thioredoxin reductase is also the reason that selenium is an essential trace element as well.[51] These enzymatic and thiol-related radical defense mechanisms are classified as endogenous defense mechanisms. Two other compounds in the body, urate and plasma albumin, are also abundant endogenous molecules that serve as sacrificial molecules much as GSH does. The difference between these molecules and GSH is that they are not regenerated and must be removed from the body when oxidized.

There are, in addition, antioxidants that are exogenous and brought into the body through the diet. These molecules become essentially sacrificial molecules that are oxidized by reactive species before other more essential biomolecules are. Vitamins C and E and carotenoids are examples of these sacrificial dietary molecules capable of scavenging ROS. While the exact biological function of vitamin E is not currently known, vitamin E can scavenge peroxyl radicals and also appears to protect membranes against lipid peroxidation by acting as a chain-breaking antioxidant.[52] As we discussed, every oxidation/reduction reaction results in formation of a new radical. The benefit derived by biological systems, when vitamins C and E are oxidized, is that the radicals produced are not highly reactive and thus easily reduced by GSH.

As we already know, plants and most animals can synthesize vitamin C. Humans are a rarity among animals that cannot. During evolution a branching occurred among primates leading to the Prosimii and the Anthropoidea suborders of monkeys. The early progenitors of humans were among the suborder anthropoidea that includes the great apes. During evolution, species acquired new genes by tandem duplication and/or polyploidization (number of chromosome sets in the nucleus),[53] and genes were sometimes lost. However, a species cannot continue to survive unless lost genes are dispensable in the environment where in which it lives. At some point in evolution early humans ingested sufficient vitamin C in their daily diets to allow continued existence, despite the loss of a critical gene involved in vitamin C biosynthesis. The ability to synthesize vitamin C in the liver requires four enzymes which convert circulating sugars into ascorbic acid (vitamin C). Humans have lost the ability to make the last enzyme, gulonolactone oxidase, in this process.[54] Nevertheless, vitamin C continues to be necessary in human metabolism because the molecule acts as a sacrificial dietary molecule in radical scavenging reactions. It is also needed in the essential reaction in oxidation of phenylalanine and tyrosine, the conversion of folacin to tetrahydrofolic acid, the synthesis of neurotransmitters dopamine, noradrenaline, and adrenaline, the synthesize of carnitine for mitochondrial energy transfer, and for collagen synthesis. The consequence of this evolutionary happenstance is that humans now require vitamin C from dietary sources.

THE ANTIOXIDANT CONTROVERSY

The bottom line of all these complex reactions is that ROS and RNS, while common in biological systems and often playing critical roles in the processes of life, can be dangerous. They are essential and yet, because of the way life evolved here on earth, they can also be lethal. Damage that radicals and reactive species can inflict on critical biomolecules must be repaired or damaged cells replaced (from stem cells) in order for organisms to continue to function. ROS and RNS-generated damage increases with age and damaging processes, such as underlying chronic inflammation, accumulated exposure to environmental injury from radiation, or xenobiotics. Simultaneously, the ability to repair or remove damaged biomolecules declines as well.[55] This imbalance between radical induced damage and the radical defense and tissue repair mechanisms has been proposed as the mechanism leading inevitably to development of age-related diseases such as cardiovascular disease, cancers, and neurodegenerative disorders.

The fact that a number of diseases are associated with oxidative stress drives the theory that antioxidants may represent an intervention strategy in these diseases. However, current evidence from clinical research has not unequivocally substantiated these theories nor demonstrated a causal role of pro-oxidants in age-related diseases. Neither has scientific evidence proved conclusively that dietary antioxidant supplementation can prevent disease or increase longevity in humans. Thus, debate and controversy has arisen among scientists, health care professionals, and the lay public alike regarding the efficacy and wisdom of using dietary antioxidant supplementation to prevent chronic diseases and delay aging.

4

WHAT DOES RESEARCH SHOW?

A dietary antioxidant is a substance in foods that significantly decreases the adverse effects of reactive oxygen species, reactive nitrogen species, or both on normal physiological function in humans.
>   —Panel on Dietary Antioxidants and Related Compounds, Food and
>   Nutrition Board, Institute of Medicine of the National Academies.

William A. Pryor, an eminent free radical and biology researcher, suggested in 2000 that a different dose-effect curve for vitamin E may exist for each disease or experimental condition and that the presence of other micronutrients has an influence on how effective vitamin E is. It is very likely that this same situation exists for every antioxidant phytochemical in our diet. Sorting out these interactions *in vivo* presents great challenges. As Pryor has stated, "there never will be a time when the science is 'complete.'"[1] To some degree, this has been the plaguing story behind the controversy and media hype surrounding antioxidants. The plethora of short popular press articles and sound bites, designed to suite the short attention spans of the busy modern day public, devotes neither time nor space for an in-depth and full explanation of the science behind antioxidants. The truth of the matter is that a living organism represents the sum total of an enormous number of complex interactions between a large number of biomolecules. This system of interactions is continually impacted by environmental conditions and complicated by the age and health of the individual. We have briefly touched upon the history of nutritional studies, but where exactly does the redox biology field stand with regard to what we know about the effects of antioxidants on health and disease?

ANTIOXIDANT RESEARCH: SYNOPSIS OF PAST AND CURRENT STUDY RESULTS

Since 1902 the Medline biomedical database has recorded over 228 thousand publications listing the keyword antioxidant(s). This number is likely an underestimate of the true number of journal articles on this subject. It is beyond the scope of this book to review the sum total of this literature; however, we can portray how our knowledge has evolved and some of the more popular current theories in the field of free radical biology and medicine. The first "antioxidant" article, cited in the Medline database, was in 1946 and the author suggested that vitamin C could be used to identify the day of ovulation.[2] The next year in which the key word "antioxidant" was cited was 1950 when suddenly 356 articles were published. Arguably, this marks the date when a relatively large number of scientists within the biomedical community began to grapple with the therapeutic validity of antioxidants and began the serious study of their involvement in radical reactions within biological systems and their possible effects on health and aging. There is no doubt that researchers had noticed health benefits of some phytochemicals much earlier; however, these phytochemicals were not yet defined as "antioxidants." Attention soon focused on these dietary phytochemicals, primarily due to their essential nature, and it was not long before studies of probable mechanisms of action were pointing in several directions. Many of these essential phytochemicals were proving to simultaneously act through multiple mechanisms. Specific primary functions were difficult to pin down. Ascorbate (vitamin C) presents a classic example of a multifunction essential phytochemical. Early studies on this vitamin began due to its critical connection to an important disease.

VITAMIN C

During the eighteenth century the British Navy was a force to be reckoned with. But this reputation came at a great cost. Sailors aboard ship for long journeys would succumb to death from the pathologic symptoms of an illness that had been known and observed for centuries—scurvy. In 1753, Dr. James Lind published his medical classic, "A Treatise of the Scurvy," wherein he described his 1740 discovery that an ounce of fresh lemon juice given each day to sailors would prevent or "clear up" the symptoms of scurvy. We now remember Dr. Lind as a great British naval physician, often referred to as "The Father of Nautical Medicine." What is less known is that after his first scientific medical experiment with twelve scorbutic sailors on shipboard, approximately 100,000 sailors died in the forty-two intervening years between Dr. Lind's recommendations to the British Admiralty and implementation of a "lime supplementation" regulation in 1795. It has been suggested that this dietary regulation was an important factor leading to Britain's "mastery of the seas," changing the course of history in the nineteenth century.

Dr. Lind and his colleagues of the day considered the abatement of symptoms as a cure of disease, which we now know was incorrect. But they did manage to recognize that scurvy was related to the foods we ate. By the end of the nineteenth century and early twentieth century, nutrition researchers had come to understand that scurvy and other diseases could be caused by "something missing" in the diet. In 1912, Casimir Funk presented his ideas regarding his hypothesis of "Vitamine-Deficiency Disease."[3] Dr. Funk discovered that beri-beri resulted from a deficiency in the diet that could be replaced by an isolated crystalline "vitamine fraction" of a yeast extract. The deficient "vitamine" was later found to be B-complex or thiamine. While Dr. Funk had coined the term "vitamine," it was Sir F. G. Hopkins who first recognized that "accessory food factors" other than carbohydrates, proteins, fats, minerals, and water were necessary for health.

Dr. Lind did not know that the active ingredient in limes and lemons responsible for preventing scurvy was ascorbate or vitamin C. Vitamin C, a water-soluble vitamin, was first isolated from the adrenal cortex and various citrus fruits by Albert Szent-Gyorgyi[4] and Charles King[5] in the late 1920s. Foods found to be rich in vitamin C were citrus fruits, tomatoes, berries, potatoes, and many other fresh vegetables (although these chemists learned early on that vitamin C was easily oxidized with extended food storage and during the process of cooking). As mentioned earlier, vitamin C can be synthesized by most animals. Guinea pigs and most primates, including humans, cannot synthesize it. It is also known that vitamin C is required in the diets of bats, at least some fish, and many birds. There are some primates that can synthesize vitamin C, but they use different organs to do so—reptiles and birds using the kidney to synthesize vitamin C and mammals and perching birds synthesizing it in the liver.[6] In animals the molecule is synthesized from glucose, while plants synthesize it from glucose and fructose.

The chemical nature of vitamin C is such that it yields electrons easily making it an excellent reducing agent and, therefore, an excellent antioxidant. In the process, as discussed previously, when vitamin C yields its electrons it becomes a radical itself. The ascorbyl radical, also known as semidehydroascorbic acid, is relatively stable and rather uncreative in biological systems. When vitamin C encounters ROS or RNS it quickly reduces them and thereby spares other molecules from potentially serious damage.

Vitamin C's electron-yielding qualities are responsible for its role as a necessary cofactor in the synthesis of collagen. In animals, vitamin C serves as a cofactor for oxygenase enzymes that incorporate oxygen into substrates. Hydroxyl groups are added to the amino acids proline or lysine in the collagen molecule by three different dioxygenase enzymes, using vitamin C as an electron donor. This reaction is necessary to produce the stable triple helix structure of collagen. It is the suboptimal operation of these enzymes that is responsible for some of the symptoms of scurvy.[7]

Other dioxygenase enzymes that require vitamin C as a cofactor are involved in tyrosine metabolism and in carnitine synthesis, a crucial molecule required to transport fatty acids into mitochondria for adenosine triphosphate (ATP) production.[8] The monooxygenases dopamine β-monooxygenase plays a role in the synthesis of norepinephrine from dopamine and can impact neurological function.[9] Peptidyl glycine α-monooxgenase modifies peptides with a terminal glycine for peptide amidation. All these enzymes are required for vitamin C to function properly.

While vitamin C's function as an enzymatic cofactor is clearly demonstrated, a large body of data exists suggesting that vitamin C can play a nonenzymatic role in redox reactions as a reducing agent both inside cells and in extracellular spaces. Frequently, we hear that vitamin C is capable of preventing low-density lipoprotein (LDL) oxidation and therefore helps prevent cardiovascular disease. Indeed, there is evidence that oxidized lipids from the LDL particle are proinflammatory and atherogenic.[10] In *ex vivo* experiments, vitamin C, vitamin E, ß-carotene, and various flavonoids inhibit metal-catalyzed LDL oxidation.[11] The mechanisms of protection *in vitro* have been proposed as radical quenching, however, observations of synergy between antioxidants suggests that the protective effects are far more complex than simple radical quenching.[12] The very relevance of metal-catalyzed oxidation in these *in vitro* and *ex vivo* LDL oxidation experiments is somewhat controversial as metals are generally well chaperoned *in vivo*. This has led to a debate among researchers regarding the "iron-heart hypothesis,"[13] first put forth by J. L. Sullivan[14] in 1981, which suggests that increased body iron stores are a risk factor for coronary heart disease (CHD). This hypothesis, which was based on markedly lower incidences of CHD in premenopausal women (who lose iron through menstruation) compared with men and postmenopausal women, is appealing and seems to be well-grounded in biochemistry. The implications were that iron depletion through phlebotomy or other means might reduce risk. While there has been inconsistent and largely negative epidemiologic evidence of the involvement of transition metal in atherosclerosis, the possible role of iron-induced lipid oxidation in atherosclerosis has not been ruled out. Indeed, subjects with thalassemia experiencing secondary iron overload resulting from continuous blood transfusions appear to have elevated levels of peroxidative damage to their cell tissues.[15] The existence of iron-induced peroxidation of lipids in this rare condition only suggests that iron-induced lipid peroxidation could contribute to lifelong injuries that possibly contribute to atherosclerosis risk among the population. It is, however, more likely that LDL oxidation *in vivo* is initiated by other events capable of producing radicals in higher quantities, such as those stemming from inflammation. Intriguingly, when animals or humans are fed dietary antioxidants, their LDLs do exhibit increased resistance to oxidation *ex-vivo*. However, the results of these experiments have sometimes been confusing. Mark McCall and Balz Frei[16] reviewed the LDL oxidation data in 1999 and concluded that with only the exception of supplemental vitamin E and possibly vitamin C lowering lipid oxidative damage in both smokers and nonsmokers, the current evidence is insufficient to conclude that antioxidant vitamin supplementation materially reduces oxidative damage in humans. This is similar to the conclusion reached by the Panel on Dietary Antioxidants and Related Compounds of the Institute of Medicine of the National Academies. McCall and Frei pointed out that the doses of vitamin E (100 mg/day) and vitamin C (1000 mg/day) that showed reduced lipid peroxidation in smokers and nonsmokers were much higher than the RDAs at the time for these vitamins (10 mg and 60 mg, respectively). Current DRIs, suggested by the Food and Nutrition Board, are also nowhere near these levels (see Appendix B). It is typical of many scientific studies that while trying to determine an effective reduction in measures of oxidative stress, they do not attempt to define an optimal dose for protection. Nor do they measure the concentrations of intervention compounds to determine whether intervention doses increase levels in the body or not.

While data is insufficient to demonstrate that antioxidants can lower oxidative damage in humans, epidemiologic data shows that dietary and supplemental intake of antioxidant vitamins is associated with a reduction in clinical measures of atherosclerosis. The Nurses' Health Study[17] and the Health Professionals' Follow-up Study[18] showed a 35 to 40 percent reduction in the incidence of major coronary events in those in the highest intake quintile for vitamin E compared to the lower intake quintile. The greatest benefit appears to be for those with vitamin E intakes between 100 and 250 IU per day. Little increase in protection was seen with higher doses of vitamin E. But there was a difference between vitamin E and vitamin C. There were no associations seen between vitamin C and vitamin E intake and major coronary events in either of these two studies. The First National Health and Nutrition Examination Survey (NHANES I) Epidemiologic Follow-up Study showed an inverse relationship between vitamin C intake (strong for males and weak for females) and for all cancers and all cardiovascular diseases.[19]

Intervention trials investigating the premise that antioxidant intake can reduce cardiovascular diseases have produced mixed results. The U.S. National Cancer Institute (NCI) and the National Public Health Institute of Finland conducted the Alpha-Tocopherol, Beta-Carotene Cancer Prevention (ATBC) Trial to determine whether vitamin supplements would prevent lung and other cancers in older male smokers. The eight-year intervention used a pill containing either 50 milligrams (mg) α-tocopherol or 20 mg of ß-carotene (as a vitamin A precursor), a combination of both, or a placebo. Vitamin E and ß-carotene were the antioxidants studied because epidemiologic studies showed high dietary intake and high serum levels of these antioxidants reduced risk of lung cancer. Interestingly, vitamin C was not included, most likely due to the lack of conclusive evidence of its anticancer association. This was unfortunate, as the ATBC Trial could easily have incorporated vitamin C and provided conclusive data regarding the efficacy of vitamin C in cancer prevention. Nevertheless, the ATBC study showed the unexpected result that ß-carotene could increase the incidence of lung cancers in smokers and that vitamin E had no effect on lung cancer incidence or overall mortality.[20] Vitamin E did, however, result in a decrease in prostate cancer cases and 41 percent fewer deaths from this cancer. In contrast, α-tocopherol intake increased the incidence of deaths from hemorrhagic stroke among men with hypertension.[21] The beta-Carotene and Retinol Efficacy Trial (CARET Study), completed in 1996, confirmed that smokers should not ingest beta-carotene supplements. This study also illustrated that there were no benefits from consumption of ß-carotene or retinol in cancer or vascular disease reduction.[22]

This study further added to the controversy about antioxidant efficacy and appeared to support the concept that antioxidants were of no benefit in disease reduction and could actually cause harm. Here again, the suite of antioxidants was limited and in this case excluded vitamin E, vitamin C, and the flavonoids. The fact that no reduction in deaths from cardiovascular causes was seen in the Physicians' Health Study among physicians who took ß-carotene supplements[23] seemed to indicate that ß-carotene was intrinsically different from other antioxidants in its health-related effects. This may be due to the fact that ß-carotene, lycopene, lutein, and other carotenoids and oxy-carotenoids (xanthophylls) are primarily effective quenchers of singlet oxygen. However, vitamin E can also quench singlet oxygen, just not as efficiently as carotenoids. But this may be debatable, as a significant role for singlet oxygen in human disease, other than those induced by radiation, is not yet established. The case-control and prospective cohort studies discussed to this point find inverse associations between the occurrence of cardiovascular disease and dietary intake of antioxidant vitamins. In contrast, however, the randomized intervention trials have either shown no benefit with ß-carotene and a possible benefit with vitamin E in cardiovascular disease. Similarly, the prospective cohort studies indicate a protective role for vitamin C against cancer. But this association was not followed up in the intervention trials mentioned thus far.

It is important to mention at this point that the observational studies that suggest antioxidants have a role in prevention of disease only examine primary prevention. In contrast, most intervention studies on antioxidant effects on disease have been aimed at secondary prevention of disease. The implication of this may be that healthy individuals consuming dietary antioxidants or supplements over long periods of time may enjoy protective effects against chronic age-related diseases including cancer, cardiovascular disease, arthritis, age-related macular degeneration and neurodegenerative diseases. But, once the etiology of a disease has occurred, antioxidants may only help to delay progression and not prevent the disease. Indeed, the same antioxidant phyto-chemical that may prevent radical-induced mutagenic lesions in DNA leading to cancer or lipid peroxidation and subsequent damage to endothelial function leading to cardiovascular disease, may be less effective in reducing the progression of these diseases. Much more research is still needed to understand the effects of antioxidants during the temporal progression of individual disease. For example, while an antioxidant may appear to have more efficacy early in the cardiovascular and cancer processes, quite a different result has been observed in the case of age-related macular degeneration (AMD), which we will discuss later.

While suboptimal levels of Vitamins C, B_{12}, B_6, and folic acid are considered by many to be factors in the development of cardiovascular disease, little research has been devoted to determining optimal levels of antioxidant nutrients. There has been considerable debate over the optimal levels of vitamin C. The RDAs, such as those for antioxidants depicted in Appendix B, are defined as "the level of intake of essential nutrients deemed to be adequate to meet the known nutritional needs of practically all healthy persons as determined by a government nutrition board upon review of all evidence based scientific data." The meaning of "adequate" is not the same as "optimal." This difference in wording is at the center of many of the disagreements regarding the usefulness of RDAs to design diets to avoid chronic illness and diseases. In the case of vitamin C, adequate levels are defined as those that prevent nutritional deficiency diseases such as scurvy in most of the population. But the public perception is that consumption of the RDA of vitamin C will lower the risk of chronic diseases such as cardiovascular disease and cancer. In recommending RDAs for vitamin C, vitamin E, selenium, and carotenoids from food (not supplements), the Food and Nutrition Board has made the effort to discriminate the needs of children, men, women, and elderly. But these categories do not indicate what may be required for individuals who do not fall into this category, including those who may be expected to have higher antioxidant requirements due to higher radical loads. Conditions known to elevate oxidative stress, which include diabetes, metabolic disorders, chronic diseases of aging, and injuries, may well consume antioxidants at higher rates and thus require higher daily intakes. Recently, nutritional science has turned more attention not only to nutrients important in preventing deficiency-related disease, but also to those nutrients and micronutrients necessary to promote optimal health.

When the discussion comes to the difference between adequate and optimal levels of vitamin C, few can speak with more expertise on the subject than Dr. Mark Levine at the NIH. Levine's group has conducted studies showing that while RDA levels of vitamin C are adequate to prevent scurvy, they may not provide the optimal levels of immunological functioning observed at higher intake levels of vitamin C.[24] Supporting this conceptual difference between adequate and optimal is the study by Gey et al., which reported that individuals with higher blood levels of antioxidant vitamins such as vitamins A, C, E, and ß-carotene had lower incidence for cancer and heart disease. These findings were from studies of people who were taking the RDA intakes of these nutrients at the time.[25] The 2000 RDAs for these nutrients were subsequently increased. However, vitamin C was still not raised to the 200 mg per day level recommended by Levine's pharmacokinetics and optimal immune system performance studies or to the 120 mg per day recommended by Carr and Frei,[26] who reviewed the literature for reduced risk of chronic diseases such as cancer, cardiovascular disease, and cataracts. The RDA for vitamin C was increased from the 60 mg per day up to 75 mg for women and 90 for men. The panel appointed by the IOM felt the scientific evidence supported a slightly higher intake level as a target for the American population, but not high enough to require anyone to take supplements or to change military or school lunch programs. On the other hand, government health authorities have strongly urged the public to consume five servings of fresh fruits and vegetables per day—an amount that would easily provide over 200 mg. of vitamin C per day.[27]

The Food and Nutrition Board suggests smokers take 125 mg per day while evidence suggests they may require 200 mg of vitamin C.[28] One report even suggests as much as 2,000 mg per day,[29] which is the upper limit (UL) set by the Food and Nutrition Board. The UL set by the Food and Nutrition Boards for vitamin C was based on the possible occurrence of diarrhea in some individuals and the premise that higher doses could be risky.

A review of the literature suggests that 4,000 mg of vitamin C is well tolerated[30] and there have even been clinical trials that have used 10,000 mg of vitamin C for several years[31] without incident. These studies show that vitamin C in high doses is safe and, indeed, these are levels that the dual Nobel Prize winner Linus Pauling and author of *The Nature of the Chemical Bond* and *Vitamin C and the Common Cold,* and *How to Live Longer and Feel Better* would have approved.

There is no doubt that there remains a continuing debate regarding supplementation versus vitamin intake from foods. There are reports, however, that seem to show benefit to vitamin C supplementation in increasing longevity[32] and decreasing risk of cataracts.[33] These benefits appear to require that tissue levels of vitamin C be elevated. Yet levels of intake higher than the RDA are required to elevate tissue vitamin C levels.[34]

The controversy regarding the IOM RDAs may all boil down to semantics, missions, and politics. The RDAs are recommendations for healthy individuals and represent minimum amounts of a nutrient that has beneficial health effects. These levels may not be optimal however. As we see have seen with vitamin C, tolerable upper levels may not be as dangerous as implied. But this is for vitamin C. Ignoring the tolerable upper limits for other vitamins and minerals, such as vitamin E and selenium, can have decidedly different consequences.

FLAVONOIDS

Flavonoids, also called bioflavonoids, are a subclass of plant polyphenols that represent over 6,000 compounds identified to date. Flavonoids are secondary metabolites that plants have conserved and diversified over a billion years of evolution.[35] These polyphenolic compounds fulfill many different functions for plants including the role of phytoalexins to protect the plant from predators and environmental stresses. Early in plant evolution flavonoids protected plants from harsh ultraviolet light and were eventually incorporated into the photosystems of plants.[36] There is even evidence that flavonoids were influential in modulating the activity of plant enzymes, growth hormones, morphogenesis, respiration, and sex determination in early plants. The ancient nature of flavonoids, and the fact that they are able to activate Rhizobium genes involved in nitrogen fixation by bacteria, suggests that this class of phytochemicals may have the potential of altering expression of mammalian genes.[37]

Plants also use flavonoids as both deterrents and attractants for insects and frugivores. During pollination they attract insects and birds by adding color to flowers by adding the anthocyanin flavonoids. Flavonoids are intrinsically bitter tasting, so color is insufficient as an attractant until it is augmented with sweet nectar as the reward to insects and birds attracted to their color. When seeds need protection, the bitter-tasting flavonoids in seed husks deter frugivores and insects until such time that the fruits are ripe. Then anthocyanins add back a color attraction to the fruits and plants and sugar is added to fruits to entice frugivores to eat them and disperse the ripe seeds. As omnivores and frugivores, humans are attracted to the aroma, color, and/or taste of fruits and berries. Many flavonoids are bioavailable and bioactive and may contribute to the health benefits associated with the consumption of fruits, vegetables, and even whole grains. But it is not just fruits that contain flavonoids. Flavonoids are ubiquitous, although in differing forms and concentrations, throughout all plant parts. So it is not unexpected that catechins, well-known flavonoids, are found in both the tender leaves of the tea plant, the fruits of the apple tree, and the root bulbs of the onion.

All flavonoids share a common structure—two or more aromatic rings linked by an oxygenated heterocyclic bridge containing one oxygen and three carbon atoms. Based on differences in their basic structures, dietary flavonoids fall into six major classes: anthocyanidins, flavanols (or catechins), flavanones, flavones, flavonols, and isoflavones. Differences in hydroxylation and methyl group placements on the ring structures define individual flavonoids within classes. One important structural point to keep in mind is the fact that, in nature, all flavonoids are linked to sugars in plant materials. Ignoring this one factor may have rendered a great deal of research on flavonoids flawed.

The isoflavones are among the first flavonoids studied biologically because their structures with hydroxyl groups in the 7 and 4′ positions of their basic ring structure provides them with an affinity to estrogen receptors. Because of this link to estrogen activity they are sometimes referred to as phytoestrogens. Another group of flavonoids, the anthocyanins, were used early in human history as dyes and thus had commercial value. Anthocyanins were extensively studied chemically, but not in regard to their biological or health-related properties. Because of their structures, the anthocyanins possess coloration ranging from oranges to deep purples. They are responsible for much of the color in plant leaves, fruits, and berries.

Another human use of flavonoids stems from the ability of some flavonoids to form polymers called tannins. The resulting plethora of hydroxyl and carboxyl groups in resulting tannin molecules make them capable of complexing with and crosslinking proteins and other macromolecules. This, as the name implies, is the fundamental process of "tanning," which fixes animal hides to produce leather.

Despite the ubiquitous presence of flavonoids in our plant-based foods, the determination of flavonoid intakes has only recently been undertaken. There are several historical reasons for this. The task of analyzing the great variety of flavonoids present in foods is challenging. Existing food databases are incomplete.

Reports estimating daily flavonoid intake at 10–100 mg often report data for only one or two of the six classes of flavonoids. In reality, such reports underestimate total flavonoid consumption. To make matters worse, flavonoid content of foods served at a meal is greatly affected by many factors, including agricultural practices, cultivated foods, ripeness, season conditions, postharvest processing, storage, and cooking.[38] Beyond all this, cultural dietary patterns and the availability of particular fruits and vegetables appear to result in dramatic differences between population groups. For example, isoflavone intake is greatest in Asian countries where soy foods are prevalent and isoflavone intake levels can reach 50 mg/d. In contrast, in the Netherlands tea is a popular beverage and this factor drives the flavanol intake levels to as much as 70 mg/d. The result is that the intake of individual foods within a specific population at any particular time of season may result in specific flavonoids disproportionately contributing to intake.

Flavonoid glycosides were once ignored by nutritional scientists because it was thought they were not absorbed. It has now been shown that some flavonoids and their metabolites can reach 10 μmol/L in plasma, which shows they are bioavailable. However, depending on the flavonoid, only 1–10 percent is absorbed.[39] Once absorbed, flavonoids do not remain in the circulation for long and most are removed from the plasma within ten hours of consumption. Few remain at low levels for over a day. Recent, research (about to be published) using studies with pigs fed blueberries in the diet suggests that anthocyanins and possibly other flavonoids may have a longer residence time in the body tissues. The differences in absorption, distribution, metabolism, and elimination between individual flavonoids vary substantially and can confound simple correlations between flavonoid intake, status, and bioactivity or health outcomes.[40]

In 1936, the Nobel Prize physiologist Szent-Gyorgyi and his colleagues first identified the ability of a lemon juice extract to decrease capillary wall permeability. They called the active ingredient "vitamin P" (latter identified as hesperidin and eriodictiol glycoside). Though flavonoids were later found nonessential and, thus, not candidates as vitamins, this early work did note a synergy between flavonoids and vitamin C and suggested their activity as antioxidants. *In vitro*, flavonoid aglycones are potent antioxidants.[41] Because of the sugar substitutions on the ring structures of flavonoids in plant materials, they become less potent as antioxidants. Little information is available on the antioxidant capacity of flavonoid phase 2 metabolite conjugates *in vitro*, though these animal metabolites predominant *in vivo* have different properties than their parent plant compounds. Hydroxyl groups on flavonoids can chelate transition minerals, such as copper and iron, to inhibit Fenton and Weiss-Haber reactions and thus inhibit generation of metal induced ROS. Some dietary flavonoids may be sufficiently effective chelators of nonheme iron in the gut and aggravate or precipitate iron-deficiency anemia.[42] As a result, flavonoids may be beneficial to people with high iron status since plasma ferritin, as has been suggested by the "iron heart theory," has been proposed as a risk factor for cardiovascular disease and also colon cancer.

Some intervention studies to lower markers of lipid and DNA oxidation and to enhance antioxidant defenses have shown positive results, and other studies have not found a significant antioxidant action of these compounds *in vivo*.[43] Such contrasting reports may reflect differences in the specific flavonoids being tested as well as differences in the health or oxidative stress status of the subjects and the dose and duration of treatment. Nonetheless, the contribution of intracellular flavonoids in quenching reactive species *in vivo* appears small relative to the higher concentration of other dietary antioxidants. In other words, based on their bioavailability and intracellular concentrations, the numbers of flavonoid molecules in the body are dramatically lower than those of glutathione, vitamin E, or vitamin C. Supplementation with 50 mg epigallocatechin gallate results in peak plasma concentrations of about 0.15 μmol/L, while the usual status of vitamin C is 3–7 mmol/L. Some synergy may exist *in vivo* between flavonoids and other components of the antioxidant defense network, including vitamins C and E, and this may have a significant impact on the quenching of reactive oxygen and nitrogen species.[44] It is much more likely, however, given the concentrations that flavonoids reach in the body, that they exert their effects indirectly by substantially increasing antioxidant defenses and redox status. Plausible mechanisms of action include induction of Phase II enzymes, which include those regulating glutathione synthetase, peroxidase,[45] and glutathione S-transferase (GST),[46] UDP-glucuronosyltransferase, NAD(P)H:quinone oxidoreductase 1 (NQO1), and epoxide hydrolase.[47]

A key factor in the bioactivity of flavonoids may be their ability to alter enzyme activity and affect cell signaling events.[48] Flavonoids have been shown to interact with all the major enzyme classes, including hydrolases, isomerases, ligases, lyases, oxidoreductases, and transferases, though the majority of these investigations have been conducted *in vitro*.[49] Flavonoids have been shown to selectively inhibit kinases by binding directly to the enzymes or to associated membrane receptors and thereby influence signal transduction pathways.[50] In other words, flavonoids can have far-reaching effects on the redox status of tissues right down at the gene level, by influencing gene expression both at the receptor and signaling levels.

FLAVONOIDS AND CHRONIC DISEASE

Research with cell cultures and animal models suggests flavonoids may play a role in promoting human health and reducing the risk of some chronic diseases. Flavonoids have been purported to have a beneficial effect on cardiovascular disease, cancer, neurodegenerative diseases, diabetes, and osteoporosis as well as having antibacterial, anticarcinogenic, antiinflammatory, diuretic, and immunostimulatory actions. Observational studies have associated the intake of flavonoids and flavonoid-rich foods with specific conditions and some acute and short-term clinical interventions indicate flavonoids can affect supposed intermediary biomarkers of chronic disease. While observational studies of the relationship between flavonoids and health represent an important research approach, they are limited due, in part, to incomplete nutrient databases and the absence of biomarkers reflecting long-term exposure. Randomized controlled trials with flavonoids examining chronic disease are slowly being undertaken.

FLAVONOIDS AND CARDIOVASCULAR DISEASE

Epidemiologic studies have found an inverse association between flavonoid intake and risk of cardiovascular disease.[51] Mechanistically, most flavonoids can increase the resistance of LDL to oxidation *in vitro*; however, *ex vivo* investigations of LDL oxidation in human studies have not proven consistent. There is a body of evidence showing that flavonoids have effects on other atherogenic mechanisms. For example, flavanols inhibit smooth muscle cell proliferation[52] and flavanones reduce blood lipids.[53] Flavonoid-rich grape juice, red wine, and coca are antithrombotic as they inhibit platelet aggregation and extend bleeding time.[54] Animal and *in vitro* studies and human intervention trials are largely consistent in showing that flavonoids can improve endothelial function and may reduce blood pressure. In human intervention trials, black tea, cocoa, red wine, and soy flavonoids promote endothelial-dependent vasodilation and improve vascular dysfunction via actions on nitric oxide production or oxidation.[55] Clearly enhancement to endothelial function could lead to improvements in blood pressure and higher intake of tea and chocolate is associated with lower blood pressure. In contrast, however, intervention studies in humans with flavonoids, especially from tea, have not been conclusive with regard to blood pressure benefits. This could be a function of the duration of these studies which tend to extend for relatively short time periods.

Flavonoid intake shows an inverse relation with cardiovascular disease in several prospective observational studies.[56] The Zutphen Elderly Study, which examined over 800 men for coronary artery disease (CAD) over a ten-year period, found high flavanol and flavone intakes were associated with significant risk reduction for cardiovascular disease.[57] The Iowa Women's Health Study followed 34,492 postmenopausal subjects for ten years as well and found that high flavonol and flavone intake reduced CAD risk.[58] Not all studies have found these associations. For example, the six-year Health Professionals Follow-up Study of 38,036 American men found no significant effect of flavonol and flavone intakes, though a reduction in coronary mortality rates was observed in those with a history of CAD.[59] A recent report was issued based on data from the Nurses' Health Study, which began in 1976. One hundred, twenty thousand female nurses between the ages of 30 and 55 were studied. Upon enrolling in the original study, 66,360 were given questionnaires about their diets in 1990, 1994, and 1998. Based on these responses, estimated intake of flavonols and flavones were made. No association was found between overall intake of flavonols and flavones in 1990 and the risk of heart attack or mortality related to heart disease over the following twelve years.[60] Another long-term twenty-eight year follow-up study from the Finnish Mobile Clinic Health Examination Survey of 9,131 people shows that higher intakes of flavonols, flavones, and flavanones were associated with a reduction in risk for incident stroke.[61]

FLAVONOIDS AND CANCER

Animal studies in rodents have demonstrated that flavonoids have anticarcinogenic efficacy in reducing the number of chemically induced tumors and the growth of implanted cancer cell lines.[62] The most probable chemopreventive mechanisms of action include modulating cytochrome P450 enzymes to prevent carcinogen activation and increasing the expression of Phase II conjugating enzymes to facilitate carcinogen excretion.[63] Some flavonoids also appear to have the capability of reducing cell proliferation by inhibiting protein kinase C and AP-1-dependent transcriptional activity to block growth-related signal transduction.[64] Yet other flavonoids can limit the initiation of cancer cells by stimulating DNA repair systems.[65]

A dozen prospective and case-control studies in Finland, the Netherlands, and the United States have found no consistent trend and association between flavonoids and cancer risk for any forms of cancer or for total cancers.[66] However, the twenty-four-year follow-up data from the Finnish Mobile Clinic Health Examination Survey of 9,959 people showed high flavonol and flavone intakes reduce risk for lung cancer for men and for women.[67] As mentioned earlier, the ATBC Cancer Prevention Study of 27,110 Finnish men, shows a significant reduction in lung cancer risk after a 6.1-year follow-up among those with the highest flavonol and flavone intake. The Iowa Women's Health Study, observing 34,651 subjects, found a decline in rectal cancer with flavanol intake that did not extend to colon cancer.[68]

FLAVONOIDS AND NEUROLOGICAL DISEASES

Some studies suggest a role for flavonoids in neurodegenerative diseases. *In vitro*, physiologically relevant concentrations of flavanols protect neuronal cells against the toxic effects of ß-amyloid, 6-hydroxydopamine, and oxidized LDL (though not H_2O_2) by modulating cell proliferation and apoptosis via increasing protein kinase C activity or inhibiting NF-κB translocation.[69] Little is known about flavonoid concentrations in the brain though it is known that their permeability across the blood-brain barrier is low.[70] Nonetheless, old rats on flavonoid-rich aqueous extracts of blueberry, spinach, or strawberry showed a reduction in age-related declines of motor behavior, cognitive function, and neuronal signal transduction, suggesting sufficient flavonoids are bioavailable and can affect brain function.[71] Grape polyphenol dietary supplementation in rats appears to protect synaptic protein functions against injury from chronic ethanol consumption.[72] Another rat study showed that epigallocatechin gallate restores dopaminergic activity following a neurotoxin induced Parkinsonian syndrome.[73] Extending into human studies, several observational studies show an inverse relationship between flavonols and flavones intake or wine consumption and the risk of age-related dementia.[74]

The difficulty with all these studies is that they are either *in vitro* with regard to mechanisms, or only investigate a few flavonoid classes *in vivo* with questionnaires to determine intake use of rather inaccurate or incomplete flavonoid databases. As we mentioned before, many factors can confound the determination of true flavonoid intake. None of these studies have investigated flavonoid supplements because they are a relatively new occurrence in the marketplace. A great deal of research has been sponsored commercially for products such as pycnogenol. Marketed as an antioxidant, pycnogenol is promoted as lowering blood pressure. Pycnogenol, made from the bark of a white pine, has been purported to be fifty times more powerful than vitamin E in its antioxidant properties and twenty times more powerful than vitamin C. These results are from *in vitro* studies. Pycnogenol is also marketed as exceptionally useful for fighting against capillary fragility and varicose veins, diabetic retinopathy, swollen legs, and other inflammatory conditions in veins and capillaries. Studied in Europe for over thirty years, pycnogenol is touted as protective against eighty different diseases, which include heart disease, cancer, arthritis, etc. Despite the body of hard science evidence that mechanisms other than radical quenching are likely responsible for flavonoid health benefit in humans, pycnogenol is still marketed as an antioxidant that "picks up" free radicals that can damage the molecular structure of human tissue.

Other "antioxidant" flavonoid supplements include Ginkgo biloba, extracts of grape seeds, bilberries, cranberries, green tea, pomegranate, and many other natural plant products. Consumers use these products in the belief they will reduce the risk of heart disease, prevent breast, prostate, and other types of cancer, lessen the chance of age-related vision problems (such as cataracts or macular degeneration), minimize the symptoms of hay fever and asthma, and fight viral infections. In most cases the science to back manufacturers' advertisements claiming of efficacy is derived from very small and very short-term corporate funded studies. While the public awaits research results supported by the NIH offices, ODS, and NCCAM, they should proceed carefully and consult the ODS Web site for recommendations.

Our knowledge of the biological actions of flavonoids is still in its infancy. *In vitro* studies suggest mechanisms of action of these compounds pertinent to health outcomes, but they are not the classic antioxidant radical quenching story. Most studies of flavonoid action have been conducted with the flavonoids that are not the metabolites actually presented to cells *in vivo*. Many flavonoids are bioavailable but achieve relatively low concentrations in the body and they are extensively metabolized both by gut microflora and body tissue. Observational studies of large cohorts have generated exciting hypotheses about the reputed health benefits of flavonoid-rich foods, however these studies are confounded both by the other ingredients in these foods and unknown interactions with other dietary and environmental factors. A great deal of research remains to be done to investigate potential antagonism or synergy when flavonoids are consumed as complex mixtures with other foods/nutrients. While many studies in humans have been published, most have been of short duration and conducted with small sample sizes, so caution is warranted when trying to extrapolate their findings to the promotion of health and prevention of disease. Still fewer studies substantially support intake of flavonoids via supplements.

VITAMIN E AND THE CAROTENOIDS

Vitamin E was discovered by Evans and Bishop in 1922.[75] However, several years earlier, these two groups of scientists began to suspect there was a missing vitamin in the nutritional needs of rodents. Semipurified diets containing vitamins A, B, C, and D could support the growth, but not reproduction in rats.[76]

A year after their first publication, Evans and Bishop conducted studies investigating reproduction in rats. They produced sterility by restricting their diets to casein, cornstarch, lard, butterfat, salt, and yeast. Soon they discovered that their missing fertility "factor X" was found in lettuce or wheat germ oil, but not in cod liver oil, flour, or wheat chaff.[77] They proceeded to isolate this essential "factor X" from plant oils. Evans and Bishop and other researchers named this "factor X" vitamin E, which was first suggested in an article by Sure.[78]

Seven years later the antioxidant properties of vitamin E were described,[79] and many consider this to be the vitamins most important biological function. Others went on to confirm vitamin E's essentiality in other animals. Soon thereafter a compound was isolated that was named α-tocopherol (from Greek offspring—tokos and, to bear—phero).[80] This name was chosen because of its vitamin E-like properties *in vivo* (restoration of fertility). In rapid succession the chemical structure of α-tocopherol was determined[81] and the molecule was synthesized.[82]

In 1946 the first *in vivo* studies were published demonstrating vitamin E's ability to protect unsaturated fatty acids from oxidation.[83] Then in some of the first vitamin deficiency studies ever conducted in primates, rhesus monkeys were placed on vitamin E deficient diets and consequences of the deficiency were fully explored.[84] Twenty seven years had passed from observation to vitamin E isolation and deficiency definition.

Physicians would accept that vitamin E was necessary for fertility. After all, this is what led to its description. As in the case of vitamin C in the Royal Navy, it would take over forty years before the concept of vitamin E's antioxidant and cardiovascular protection properties would even be discussed among cardiologists. Physicians of the time knew very little about vitamins and their functions and even less about free radical biology.

As we know well in this day and age, vitamins are considered essential when deficiency symptoms develop in their absence. Vitamin E deficiencies are most often seen in individuals who cannot absorb dietary fat or have fat metabolism disorders (such as abetalipoproteinemia), Crohn's disease, pancreatic insufficiency, or liver disease. Deficiencies may also manifest themselves as neurological abnormalities and require vitamin E as a course of therapy. Symptoms of vitamin E deficiency include muscle weakness, poor nerve impulse transmission, and retinopathies.

While vitamin E was discovered nearly eighty-five years ago,[85] a clear biological function has still not emerged from the research despite clear evidence of deficiency symptoms. Vitamin E, to some extent, is a vitamin in search of a disease. We know vitamin E has physiologically important antioxidant properties, but evidence continues to emerge showing non-antioxidant effects in cellular metabolism. As an antioxidant, vitamin E is an effective chain-breaking antioxidant, preventing the propagation of free radical damage in biological membranes and plasma lipoproteins. It effectively quenches peroxyl radicals, thereby protecting polyunsaturated fatty acids against lipid peroxidation. Vitamin E also appears to limit the oxidation of LDL-cholesterol[86] and has cardioprotective capabilities because it inhibits platelet aggregation and enhances vasodilation. Its mechanistic actions also extend to influences in signal transduction by inhibiting protein kinase C and these effects may further influence inflammatory and immune responses.[87] Enhancing immune function is proposed as one mechanism whereby vitamin E may protect against cancers.[88]

What exactly is vitamin E? Natural vitamin E is a group of eight different isomers that include four tocopherols and four tocotrienols. All have a chromanol ring that has a hydroxyl group capable of donating a hydrogen atom to reduce free radicals. The molecule has a hydrophobic (phytyl tail) side chain that allows it to be inserted into biological membranes much as fatty acids are. Both the tocopherols and tocotrienols have alpha, beta, gamma, and delta forms that are differentiated by the number of methyl groups on the chromanol ring. These substitutions on the chromanol ring determine the biological activity of each form.

Because of its history of discovery as essential to fertility in rats, the measure of "vitamin E" activity is based on fertility enhancement by the prevention of spontaneous abortions in pregnant rats and is relative to α-tocopherol and expressed in international units (IU). Alpha-tocopherol is the most active form of vitamin E in humans. One IU of vitamin E is defined as the biological equivalent of 0.667 milligrams of the isomeric form RRR-alpha-tocopherol. One IU of vitamin E is also equivalent to 1 milligram of all-rac-alpha-tocopheryl acetate, the commercially available form commonly used in dietary supplements.

Tocopherols have a saturated (no double bonds) phytyl tail. When there are double bonds present in this tail, the molecules are then called tocotrienols and four tocotrienols exist having ring structures equivalent to the four tocopherols. Vitamin E supplements can contain chemically synthesized vitamin E, "d, l-alpha-tocopherol" (usually found in supplements as the acetate ester), extracted vitamin E esters from natural sources, or highly purified fractions of extracted natural d-alpha tocopherol. Because of the manufacturing process, synthetic vitamin E is a mixture of left- and right-handed stereoisomers of a chiral molecule alpha tocopheryl acetate and only one-eighth of its production is actually the isomeric form RRR-alpha tocopherol. This is the reaason that synthetic vitamin E is not as active as the natural alpha-tocopherol form. The full health implications of this fact is not completely known. We only know that synthetic vitamin E is considered by many to be less effective in combating cardiovascular disease and cancers.

In the production of natural extracted vitamin E, the process becomes much more economical if the vitamers (defined as one of two or more closely related chemicals that fulfill the same specific vitamin function) are converted into d-alpha tocopheryl acetate or d-alpha tocopheryl succinate by esterification and methylation. Unfortunately, human absorption of tocopheryl esters is less efficient than it is in rats.[89] This results in lower bioavailability and less activity than anticipated in humans. A second problem in production of natural extracted E is encountered by premature babies, patients suffering illness, and the elderly who cannot de-esterify tocopheryl acetates or tocopheryl succinates as effectively as healthy humans.

The Institute of Medicine (IOM) established the RDA for vitamin E on the basis of available alpha-tocopherol evidence as this is considered to be the most biologically relevant tocopherol. The IOM suggests that men and women consume 15 mg vitamin E per day (equivalent to 22.5 IU) and determined that most North American adults get enough vitamin E from their normal diets to meet current recommendations. The NHANES III (1988–1991) and the CSFII (1994) national food studies indicated, however, that most American diets do not provide the recommended intakes of vitamin E. The IOM counters that because fats are underreported in national surveys and because the kind and amount of fat added during cooking is often not known, these national surveys underestimate actual vitamin E intakes.

The IOM established an UL for vitamin E at 1,000 mg (1,500 IU) per day based on animal study evidence because vitamin E can act as an anticoagulant and may increase the risk of bleeding problems.[90] Little is known about the long-term safety of vitamin E supplementation and studies investigating vitamin E supplement safety have been for short periods of time, often less than a year. Meydani[91] found beneficial results when long-term doses of vitamin E supplements were given to healthy older adults. In his study, he investigated the long-term effect of vitamin E supplement doses consisting of 60, 200, or 800 IU for 235 days. All three doses improved immune function. The study concluded that 200 IU per day was the optimal amount of vitamin E for increased immune response in elderly populations. More than 40 percent of older Americans currently have a vitamin E intake below the RDA.

Considering that the best dietary sources of vitamin E are nuts, seeds, oils, and whole grains, it would be difficult to reach a daily intake of 200 IU from diet alone. So, this leaves us with the question: should a vitamin E supplement be taken in addition to a healthy diet as the best approach to "optimal health"? Many think so and some take supplements over 200 IU/day in the false belief that more is better.

Miller et al.[92] published their results of a meta-analysis in 2005, investigating high dose vitamin E trials ($\geq$ 400 IU). These trials studied vitamin E in relation to risk with patients already at high risk for cardiovascular disease (CVD). The findings seemed disturbing because the results showed statistically significant, although small, increased risk of all-cause mortality reported among those subjects taking a vitamin E supplement. This news circulated quickly among physicians who promptly advised their patients to stop taking vitamin E supplements and vitamin E supplement sales dropped dramatically from previous levels. The results of this study highlight the power of bad news. Vitamin E sales have continued to be depressed from previous high levels even after three more published meta-analyses of vitamin E trials found that vitamin E supplementation doses up to 800 IU were *not* associated with all-cause or cardiovascular mortality.[93]

In 2005, Hathcock et al.[94] reviewed the literature, including twenty studies, and concluded that the evidence that high vitamin E intakes were harmful to humans was not convincing. This evidence was from a clinical trial using vitamin E supplements in amounts less than or equal to 1,600 IU. For now, vitamin E supplement levels below the IOM's established UL for vitamin E is at 1,000 mg (1,500 IU) per day and appears to be safe.

VITAMIN E AND CARDIOVASCULAR DISEASE

Observational studies have associated lower rates of heart disease with higher vitamin E intake. These studies held promise that vitamin E was protective against coronary heart disease.[95] A study of 87,245 female nurses suggested that high intake of vitamin E from diet and supplements was associated with between 30 percent and 40 percent lower incidence of heart disease and that this was due primarily to vitamin E supplementation rather than intakes from food.[96] Similarly, a reduction in heart disease-related mortality was observed in men and women in a smaller Finnish study.[97] Intervention studies were undertaken to investigate these relationships. The Women's Angiographic Vitamin and Estrogen (WAVE) trial[98] found no effects from supplements providing 400 IU vitamin E and 500 mg vitamin C twice a day in 423 postmenopausal women. One of the larger studies, the Heart Outcomes Prevention Evaluation (HOPE) Study, followed 10,000 patients at high risk for heart attack or stroke over 4.5 years and supplemented them with 265 mg (400 IU) of vitamin E daily. No effect was found. A follow-up study will determine if a longer intervention with vitamin E supplements will alter this outcome.[99]

VITAMIN E AND CANCER

Human studies investigating the relationship between vitamin E intake and cancer have been inconclusive. In the Finnish Alpha-Tocopherol, Beta-Carotene Cancer Prevention (ATBC) Study, α-tocopherol supplementation decreased prostate cancer incidence, whereas beta-carotene increased the risk of lung cancer and total mortality.[100] Higher intake of vitamin E has also been associated with decreased incidence of breast cancer in some studies, while others show no relationship.[101] However, some believe that vitamin E isomers, for example gamma-tocopherol, and other nutrients such as selenium, may be responsible for reduced incidence of prostate cancer.[102] When the effect of dietary factors, including vitamin E, on reducing the risk of developing breast cancer was examined in over 18,000 postmenopausal women in New York State, vitamin E had no influence.[103]

The Iowa Women's Health Study provided evidence that an increased dietary intake of vitamin E may decrease the risk of colon cancer.[104] On the other hand, the Nurses' Health Study and the Health Professionals Follow-up Study found no association between vitamin E intake and risk of colon cancer.[105] A large study of 1,000,000 adults in the United States found that over the long term (more than ten years), supplementation with vitamin E was associated with a reduced risk of death from bladder cancer while the same association was not seen from vitamin C supplements.[106] The Prostate, Lung, Colorectal, and Ovarian Cancer Screening Trial (PLCO Trial), conducted in 29,361 male smokers, found that vitamin E supplementation was associated with reduced risk of advanced prostate cancer.[107] The ATBC and PLCO findings appear to suggest that vitamin E supplementation may benefit individuals who may experience elevated oxidative stress or elevated immune stress, such as smokers. One interesting observation in the ATBC study showed that vitamin E supplementation resulted in fewer occurrences of acute viral nasopharyngitis (commonly known as the common cold) among some smokers.[108] Again, this may be a function of vitamin E's ability to enhance immune function rather than any antioxidant function.

VITAMIN E AND VISION

Age-related macular degeneration and cataracts are leading causes of vision loss among aging individuals worldwide. Observational studies have found that lens opacity, an early sign of cataract formation, was lessened in subjects who took vitamin E supplements regularly.[109] Under conditions of oxidative stress, which has been conclusively demonstrated to exist in smokers, vitamin E supplementation may not be sufficient to delay cataract formation.[110] The Age Related Eye Disease Study (AREDS) was designed to test the efficacy of long-term dietary supplementation in preventing age-related macular degeneration (AMD). Results of the AREDS provided some evidence that antioxidants, vitamins and minerals, may be effective in preventing or treating AMD. This study focused on the effects of a combination of antioxidant vitamins A, C, and E and zinc on the development of cataracts and AMD. The results showed some protective effect of antioxidant supplements in preventing the progression of moderately advanced cases of dry macular degeneration or in preventing vision loss in individuals with unilateral wet macular degeneration.[111] The overall findings of the AREDS study regarding antioxidant supplementation were published in the AREDS report No. 8.[112] In contrast to the AREDS findings, another randomized trial of 1,193 subjects reported that after four years of supplementation, 500 IU per day of vitamin E had little benefit in reducing the risk of development or progression of AMD.[113] The suggestion has been offered by AREDS investigators that, as in the AREDS study, too few of the subjects in this study progressed to advanced AMD. Indeed, at present this study may validate the AREDS finding that antioxidant vitamins, at the tested dose, appear to be of little benefit in the early stages of AMD. But there is the possibility they may be helpful in preventing the advanced stages that develop with inclusion of inflammatory processes.

Although it was noted that mortality in AREDS was half that observed in the general population, AREDS was not able to unequivocally prove the safety of high-dose antioxidant supplementation. This may be due to the fact that the typical volunteer for this study was healthy and mobile. The dose of vitamin C (500 mg) used in the formulation was approximately five times what the general population receives from diet alone. The 400-IU dose of vitamin E was approximately thirteen times the RDA while the dose of zinc, as zinc oxide, was approximately five times the RDA. These levels of zinc and vitamins C and E can usually be obtained only by supplementation.

VITAMIN E AND NEUROLOGICAL FUNCTION

Among other health indicators, the Iowa Women's Health Study monitored the cognitive function of subjects during the study and in a four-year follow-up study.[114] Five and a half years after commencement of vitamin E or placebo intervention, 6,377 subjects were tested for their performance across five cognitive tests. The combined data showed no significant differences in cognition. However, there were trends evident that were non-significant that suggested, among the lower intake levels, there may be some benefit in staving off age related cognitive decline with supplementation.

CAROTENOIDS

Carotenoids are among the most ubiquitous of natural pigments comprising over 600 fat-soluble phytochemicals. They have been the focus of research efforts in the fields of chemistry, biochemistry, physiology, nutrition, and medicine for over a century. In 2005 Norman Krinsky and Elizabeth J. Johnson wrote a review of carotenoid actions and their relation to health and disease, citing over 300 references. This represents only a portion of the research that has been devoted to carotenoids and their effects on human health.[115] Like the flavonoids, carotenoids are a large family of compounds. Fortunately for health researchers, only about two dozen appear to be retained in the tissues of humans and only two, lutein and zeaxanthin, are found in the retina and lens of the eye. Lutein and zeaxanthin are classified as xanthophylls and β-carotene and lycopene are carotenes. Together, because of their important biological functions in humans, they are the most studied of the carotenoids. Alpha-carotene, β-carotene, and beta-cryptoxanthin can be converted into retinol and thus used directly for photoreception.[116] However, most of the other carotenoids can't be converted into retinol in humans. Thus, they are not involved in retinol related functions. Lutein and zeaxanthin also cannot be converted to retinol. However, they are specifically deposited in the macular region of the retina. The exact reason for such specific deposition in human retina is not known but there are theories including antioxidant function in protection from photo-induced damage.[117]

The health beneficial properties of carotenoids are attributed in part to their antioxidant activity, however, as we have seen for other antioxidants, other protective mechanisms are likely. One example is the role of lutein and zeaxanthin as light filters in the retina and lens, absorbing damaging blue light that is thought to be responsible for damage leading to age-related macular degeneration and cataracts.

Perhaps more than other antioxidant phytochemical, attention has been paid to the pro-oxidant capabilities of carotenoids.[118] While it is clear carotenoids are antioxidants *in vitro,* and many feel they are antioxidants *in vivo* as well,[119] there are some who feel the *in vivo* data does not substantiate this status.[120] *In vitro* carotenoids are best known for their ability to quench singlet excited oxygen and therefore they should be excellent *in vivo* antioxidants protecting against photosensitized oxidations.[121] Carotenoids, added directly by supplement or eaten as foods, are able to protect LDL from oxidation *in vivo* or *ex vivo.*[122] But even these studies are not providing consistent results as some studies have shown that some carotenoids can actually increase LDL oxidation.[123] A study that demonstrated that LDL composition does not predict resistance to Cu-stimulated oxidation, and that LDL from volunteers in countries with lower rates of CVD do not necessarily have greater resistance to oxidation, have brought into question the concept that enhancing the carotenoid content of LDL can, by itself, have an impact on LDL resistance to oxidation.[124]

Animal studies are complicated by the fact that most animals absorb carotenoids very poorly. Ferrets, gerbils, and preruminant calves are among the animals that absorb carotenoids, however, relatively few antioxidant studies have been conducted with in these animals.[125] As a result, studies to determine the effectiveness of carotenoids as antioxidants must be conducted in humans where dietary carotenoids are well absorbed.[126] According to Rice-Evans et al.,[127] the evidence that carotenoids are antioxidants *in vivo* is not very convincing. Indeed, despite numerous studies of the effects of carotenoid supplementation in humans on levels of malondialdehyde, a marker of lipid oxidation or 8-hydroxy-2'-deoxyguanosine (8OHdG), a marker of DNA oxidation, have not conclusively shown antioxidant activity *in vivo*. There is a body of literature concerning the observation that under high oxygen tension, β-carotene can become oxidized and become a pro-oxidant and this literature has been reviewed by Palozza.[128]

Findings of the ATBC study in humans that showed increased lung cancer in β-carotene-supplemented smokers generated inquiry into the phenomenon. Cigarette smoke is known to be a pro-oxidant. The theory was presented that high concentrations of β-carotene could be oxidatively destroyed by cigarette smoke creating oxidized metabolites that could favor carcinogenesis.[129] Indeed this appears to be the case, however not all carotenoids behave the same. Lycopene appeared to protect ferrets against smoke-induced lung carcinogenesis.[130]

CAROTENOIDS AND HUMAN STUDIES

The concept that carotenoids, by their capacity to trap peroxyl radicals and quench singlet oxygen are cardioprotective, appears to be borne out in observational epidemiological studies of the effects of carotenoid-rich foods on CVD.[131] Supporting this concept is a study that 3,254 people followed from 1989 to 1995, which showed that higher serum levels of carotenoids with pro-vitamin A activity significantly reduces the risk of mortality from cardiovascular disease and colorectal cancer.[132] The Survey in Europe on Nutrition and the Elderly in 1,168 elderly men and women followed for ten years showed that plasma carotene concentrations were associated with a 21 percent lower mortality risk for every 0.39 micromol/L increase in plasma carotene, a 41 percent lower mortality risk for cancer, and a 17 percent lower risk of mortality due to cardiovascular disease.[133] Data obtained from the Nurses' Health Study show that dietary intake of the antioxidant carotenoids α- and ß- carotene are inversely associated with coronary artery disease.[134] Women whose consumption of ß-carotene was the highest had a 26 percent lower risk of developing coronary artery disease than women whose intake was lowest in the group. The Lipid Research Clinic's Coronary Primary Prevention Trial and Follow-up Study (LRC-CPPT) found that participants with higher serum carotenoid levels had a decreased risk of coronary heart disease.[135] This finding was stronger among men who never smoked. A study of 748 cases and 1,411 hospital and community controls in four Latin American countries evaluated the association between certain elements of diet and invasive cervical cancer.[136] This study found a reduced risk of cervical cancer associated with higher intakes of vitamin C, ß-carotene, and other carotenoids. The results are consistent with those of other investigations and provides support for a protective effect of vitamin C, carotenoids, and other substances found in the same fruits and vegetables against the development of invasive cervical cancer.

Among the intervention trials, as mentioned above, the Alpha-Tocopherol Beta-Carotene (ATBC) Trial, a large randomized trial conducted between 1985 and 1993, tested the effects of 50 mg/d α-tocopherol and/or 20 mg/d ß-carotene on more than 29,000 male smokers. The ATBC trial was abruptly stopped after adverse trends including lung cancer were observed among its test subjects.

In contrast, the Physicians' Health Study found ß-carotene supplementation over a thirteen-year period in healthy men produced neither benefit nor harm.[137] The investigators suggest the results demonstrated that β-carotene alone was not responsible for the health benefits seen among people who ate plenty of fruits and vegetables.

A study of 413 nonsmokers in New York State, from 1982 to 1985, suggests that while vitamin E supplements reduce the risk of lung cancer in nonsmoking men and women, this relationship also exists for ß-carotene from dietary sources, that is, raw fruits and vegetables.[138] Reports from many studies have suggested that carotenoids, and in particular lycopene, could be cancer preventive agents. However, in a large prospective study—the Prostate, Lung, Colorectal, and Ovarian Cancer Screening Trial of 844 subjects followed over an eight-year period—lycopene and other carotenoids were found unrelated to prostate cancer. High serum ß-carotene concentrations were also associated with increased risk for aggressive, clinically relevant prostate cancer.[139]

In 1996 the Carotene and Retinol Efficacy Trial (CARET), a large study of 18,000 current and former male and female smokers and asbestos-exposed males, found that the dietary supplement ß-carotene and retinol (vitamin A) increased lung cancer risk. Participant risk remained increased even after they stopped supplementation, especially in women and former smokers.[140] Principal researchers in CARET believe that ß-carotene may change the metabolism of estrogen, which can be involved in carcinogenesis.

A group of 864 patients, supplemented with placebo; ß-carotene (25 mg daily); vitamin C (1 g daily) and vitamin E (400 mg daily); or ß-carotene plus vitamins C and E was studied for development of new adenomas by complete colonoscopic examinations at one and four years after entering the study. No evidence that either ß-carotene or vitamins C and E reduced the incidence of adenomas argued against the use of supplemental ß-carotene and vitamins C and E to prevent colorectal cancer. The investigators state that while their data do not prove definitively that these antioxidants have no anticancer effect, other dietary factors may make more important contributions to the reduction in the risk of cancer associated with a diet high in vegetables and fruits.[141]

Several years later these same investigators undertook another study of the effect of ß-carotene on colorectal cancer. A total of 864 subjects who had had an adenoma removed and were polyp-free were randomly assigned to the same treatments of the previous study, and were followed with colonoscopy for adenoma recurrence one year and four years after the qualifying endoscopy. This time smoking and alcohol use data was collected. A study was made of the effects of ß-carotene on adenoma recurrence. The results showed that supplementation with ß-carotene was beneficial among subjects who did not drink or smoke, but risk was increased among those who drank and/or smoked. However, alcohol intake and cigarette smoking appear to modify the effect of ß-carotene supplementation on the risk of colorectal adenoma recurrence.[142]

CAROTENOID CONCLUSIONS

There are over 850 studies assessing the effects of antioxidant supplements. A great many of these studies show that carotenoids lower the risk of diseases. The media and public have drawn the conclusion that taking carotenoid supplements is safe and effective if adequate amounts are not obtained from dietary sources. But then there is confusion whenever dire warnings are issued by the media in response to reports such as that from the CARET study. What is missing in public perception of carotenoids is that the vast majority of evidence indicating beneficial effects of carotenoids are seen when they are consumed as a mixture of carotenoids and in the company of sufficient amounts of other antioxidants such as vitamin E, C, and selenium. Carotenoids are beneficial as part of the antioxidant defense system but in high concentrations and alone they appear to be unstable and when oxidized they form dangerous radicals that may themselves promote cancer development in the body.

SELENIUM

Jöns Jakob Berzelius, a Swedish chemist, who is considered to be one of the founders of modern chemistry, with his lab students discovered a number of elements including silicon, cerium, lithium, vanadium, thorium, and selenium. Berzelius also was trained as a medical doctor and, therefore, had an interest in biology where he first defined the distinction between organic compounds (those containing carbon) and inorganic compounds. But he also realized early on that many inorganic elements were contained within or associated with "inorganic molecules." Colaborating with a Dutch organic chemist, Gerhardus Johannes Mulder, they analyzed these inorganic elements in organic compounds. Berzelius suggested the term "protein" to Mulder when describing a class of (very large) organic molecules that appeared to have a common empirical formula. Berzelius thought that proteins were the primitive substance of animal nutrition that plants manufactured for the herbivores.

One of the elements Berzelius discovered in 1817, selenium, was found in association with tellurium. Tellurium, discovered in 1782 by Hungarian chemist Franz-Joseph Müller von Reichenstein (Müller Ferenc), was named by Martin Heinrich Klaproth who succeeded in isolating it. Tellurium was derived from the Latin *tellus* meaning "earth." The association of selenium with tellurium led to its name, which was based on the Greek *selene* meaning

"Moon." Selenium has had many industrial applications throughout history, but is also important in biology.

Selenium is found in many plants and thought to be utilized as a defense mechanism against being eaten by herbivores. Animals that consume some plants growing in locations where selenium soil concentrations exceed 2 ppm can become poisoned over time. Some plants appear to require selenium for growth while others do not. Animal toxicity has been described based on livestock symptoms including blind staggers or alkali disease. Blind staggers, the more serious symptom, occurs within weeks of livestock consuming plants growing in high soil selenium locations. Alkali disease develops over months in animals grazing on plants in high selenium soils that contain levels (5 to 40 ppm) of selenium. Although he did not know of the element, Marco Polo was one of the first to write about selenium toxicity in the thirteenth century. He noticed while in western China that the sloughing off of the hooves of horses was associated with their consumption of certain plants in the regions. Today we know he was describing selenium toxicity based on his location, which has soils that contain the highest concentrations of selenium in the world. In humans, intake of selenium less than 900 micrograms daily (for adults) is unlikely to cause adverse reactions. Prolonged intakes of selenium, at doses of 1,000 micrograms (or one milligram) or greater daily, may cause adverse reactions that are first manifest as garlic-like breath odor, fatigue, irritability, skin rash, nausea, and vomiting. Eventually hair loss and fingernail blackening and loss will occur as it did in Marco Polo's horses. The Food and Nutrition Board has recommended the following Tolerable Upper Intake Levels (UL) for selenium at 400 micrograms/d and noted that the Lowest-Observed-Adverse-Effects-Level (LOAEL) for adults is about 900 micrograms daily.

But there is another side to selenium in animals. Although it is toxic in large doses, selenium is an essential micronutrient for animals. This became strikingly clear in the 1970s when a potentially fatal cardiomyopathy disorder, known as Keshan disease and rampant in humans in certain areas of China, was linked to dietary selenium deficiency. It seems that China has regions that contain some of the world's most selenium-poor and selenium-rich soils. Because of this discovered link, Keshan disease can now be prevented and treated, should it occur, with selenium supplementation.

Similarly another disease, "big joint disease," is found in the selenium-poor regions of Tibet, Siberia, North Korea, and China. This disease, Kashin-Beck disease, is an osteoarthropathy and manifests itself as atrophy, degeneration, and necrosis of cartilage tissue.

Selenium deficiency is also found to produce symptoms of hypothyroidism, including goitre, extreme fatigue, mental decline, cretinism, and recurrent miscarriage. It was discovered that selenium was essential to the functioning of the enzyme iodothyronine deiodinases (thyroid hormone deiodinases). Iodothyronine deiodinases are responsible for converting the inactive form of thyroid hormone (thyroxine or T_4) to biologically active thyroid hormone (triiodothyronine or T_3).[143] Three different selenium-dependent iodothyronine deiodinases exist that can both activate and inactivate thyroid hormone. All require selenium for proper function, thus selenium is an essential element in the regulation of thyroid hormones leading to functional metabolism and normal growth and development.[144]

While low selenium levels in soils grow low selenium content plant foods and can present a risk to populations dependent on these foods, selenium deficiency is relatively rare today in healthy well-nourished individuals. Part of this is due to the large-scale distribution of foods nationally and internationally. There are, however, medical conditions where selenium deficiencies do occur and are primarily seen in patients with severely diminished intestinal function and those undergoing total parenteral nutrition (TPN). The Food and Nutrition Board, based on all these factors, recommended that the AI and RDA for selenium for healthy adults are 55 micrograms per day.

SELENIUM ANTIOXIDANT ACTIONS

As we already discussed, selenium itself is not a direct radical quencher. It is necessary for the proper function of the selenoproteins, many of which are important components in the endogenous antioxidant defense system. Selenium functions as a cofactor to the glutathione peroxidases that catalyze the reaction using GSH to reduce hydrogen peroxide to water. It also reduces lipid peroxides to the corresponding alcohols. Similarly the selenoprotein enzymes, thioredoxin reductases, reduce intramolecular disulfide bonds and regenerate vitamin C from its oxidized state.

SELENIUM IN CARDIOVASCULAR DISEASE

There is strong evidence that meeting the RDA for selenium prevents Keshan disease. In relation to cardiovascular disease causes, epidemiological data shows an inverse relationship between blood selenium levels and increased rates of heart disease found in low-selenium areas.[145]

Prospective studies investigating the relationship between selenium intake or plasma levels and heart disease have been inconclusive, although two studies conducted in Finland found an association. However, selenium intake has been historically very low in Finland.[146] In contrast, studies in populations with higher selenium intakes have found no association between selenium intake or plasma levels and cardiovascular disease.[147]

This has led some to speculate that only very low selenium levels have a relationship to risk of cardiovascular disease.[148] As yet, controlled prevention trials to investigate selenium alone in prevention and therapy of cardiovascular disease have not been completed.

SELENIUM IN CANCER

Study data continue to show that low dietary intake of selenium is associated with increased incidence of lung, colorectal, skin, and prostate cancers. In countries and locations where selenium intakes are low, a higher rate of cancer deaths is reported.[149] Additionally, case-control studies show that patients suffering from cancers have lower circulating concentrations of selenium.[150] It is known that as diseases progress, blood levels of selenium decline. Again, in Finland where selenium levels have been low, the large Finnish Mobile Health Examination Survey showed a reduced risk of cancers in men taking supplements, predominantly lung and stomach cancers.[151] Inverse associations have also been noted between selenium status and risk of colorectal adenomas[152] and prostate cancer.[153]

Evidence from intervention trials, such as the randomized controlled trials conducted in Linxian, China (again in a region with historically low selenium soils and where local grown foods are depended upon), show that supplementation with a combination of ß-carotene, selenium, and vitamin E lowers the incidence of total cancer mortality, particularly stomach cancers.[154] How much of this reduction is due to selenium is unclear. Another study, also conducted in China in the town of Qidong, supplemented diets with selenium-fortified salt and showed reductions in liver cancer risk.[155] But the population of Qidong suffered an increased rate of other cancers and hepatitis B infections.[156]

A recently reviewed body of literature related to selenium and its influence on viral pathogenicity suggests that the effect of host nutrition on viral disease via oxidative stress, immune dysfunction, and increased viral pathogenicity must now include the ability of the virus to mutate under conditions of oxidative stress.[157] More research is required to understand the relationship between antioxidants, viral pathogenicity, and cancers. Some of these relationships may account for the observations found in Qidong and other studies that find a relationship between selenium and liver cancer reductions.

The largest intervention trial conducted to date, Nutritional Prevention of Cancer Trial, investigated the relationship between high selenium intake and cancer protection. One thousand, three hundred and twelve subjects in the United States who had a previous history of skin cancer were studied.[158] Results showed that supplementation with 200 mg selenium/d reduced the risk of total cancer incidence and mortality. In this study selenium did not prevent the recurrence of skin cancer, but did reduce the incidence of lung, colorectal, and prostate cancers. Here again there was evidence that at least for prostate cancer, the benefits of selenium supplementation appeared to accrue to those who had low plasma selenium levels on admission to the study.[159] The implication is that selenium may be more effective in preventing cancer than in stopping progression.

The Selenium and Vitamin E Cancer Prevention Trial (SELECT) in the United States investigated the link between selenium and vitamin E supplementation and risk of prostate cancer. The SU.VI.MAX study, investigating lower dose supplementation using a multivitamin combination (vitamins C, E, ß-carotene) and minerals (selenium and zinc) are currently underway. Early results look promising for men, but not for women. At this time in the United Kingdom a large intervention trial is being established to investigate prevention of cancer by intervention with selenium. The Prevention of Cancer by Intervention with Selenium (PRECISE) will supplement subjects for five years with different doses of selenium and study the incidence of cancer in a normal healthy population.

CONCLUSIONS FROM SELENIUM STUDIES

Studies to date indicate low selenium level is not, in itself, carcinogenic. But it does appear to increase susceptibility to malignancy in the presence of carcinogens. Studies seem to show that selenium, in adequate amounts, is useful in preventing some cancers but not in stopping them once they develop. These are only preliminary conclusions and, as noted, research is underway to confirm this speculation. There is as yet no strong evidence that additional selenium supplementation in those with already adequate diets have protective benefits for either cardiovascular disease or cancers. Again, the evidence suggests that for those who are ill or immune compromised, there may be benefits to supplementation. However, unlike vitamin C and vitamin E, selenium supplemented at levels equal to or higher than 900 micrograms daily can be toxic.

WHAT SHOULD WE CONCLUDE FROM ALL THIS

Although this is not an exhaustive review of all the antioxidant and health literature, and there are many studies we did not discuss, we feel these are the most important. What we hope we have achieved is to provide a general sense for the concepts that antioxidants are essential, are safe when obtained from foods, and are generally safe when used conservatively as supplements. However, there is much more research that remains to be completed before optimal levels for these nutrients can be established.

There are also dangers to extreme supplementation. Oxidative stress is implicated in the pathogenesis of many degenerative diseases, including cardiovascular disease, cancer, AMD, cataracts, and neurodegenerative diseases. In *in vitro* and animal studies, antioxidants (including vitamins E, C, β-carotene, and flavonoids) show antioxidant activity and plausible mechanisms of action in biological systems. This is especially so in *ex vivo* lipoproteins and cell culture experiments. Observational studies consistently show a relationship between diets rich in antioxidant-containing fruits and vegetables and reduced risk for chronic diseases such as cancer and heart disease. However, despite this evidence, clinical trials of single antioxidant micronutrient supplementation, and some multivitamin supplements, continue to show inconclusive results. In most of these studies, results either show an effect or are null with regard to efficacy. Very few studies, the ATBC and CARET studies most notorious among them, have shown harm from supplementation. The probable reason for the toxic effects of carotenoids in smokers in the CARET study is that at high levels these antioxidants are oxidized to carotenoid radical species that, unlike tocopherol and ascorbate radicals, are not recycled or effectively rendered harmless.[160]

Supplementing the diet with vitamin C or vitamin E may have beneficial effects for some individuals who are either suffering from certain malabsorption conditions or under oxidative stress due to illness or advancing age. But for the majority of people supplementing at levels below the IOM upper tolerable limits, the worst they will suffer is loss of the funds required to purchase these supplements. If they experience only peace of mind, then there may yet be benefits we cannot measure. Science is difficult to compare given the many variables across studies. Nevertheless, there seems to be a difference emerging with regard to the efficacy of antioxidant nutrients in primary versus secondary disease prevention.

Among the antioxidant supplements very little is known about the flavonoids, perhaps because there are so many and they enjoy so many potential mechanisms of action. Yet, it is precisely this lack of knowledge that presents a danger with regard to safety. Flavonoids are the most drug-like molecules among the "antioxidants." When claims are made that the contents of a bottle can aid in treating over eighty diseases, one must wonder about the validity of the claims. If claims are too good to be true, then chances are good they are not. On the other hand, flavonoids may represent the critical components in the antioxidant mix to achieve the efficacy of fruits and vegetables. A saving grace with regards to their safety may be in their very low bioavailability and the fact that the body treats them as xenobiotic compounds.

A couple of meta-analysis show that extreme levels of vitamin E intake may increase mortality[161] while another shows all antioxidants cause increased risk of all morality.[162] These studies have generated much concern among both the media and public. Yet this upheaval is the direct result of studies presented to the public before respected scientists in the field are able to add their assessment of the quality or meaning of these analyses. Science has operated for generations on consensus based on debate of the evidence. The media love a controversy because it sells magazines and newspapers. The safety of vitamins C and E, and selenium are established. The tolerable upper levels (UL) established by the Food and Nutrition Board (vitamin E at 1,500 IU, vitamin C at 2,000 mg, and selenium at 400 μg) are conservative estimates. When considering mega doses of any phytochemical, a person essentially becomes a biological explorer with all the risks implied therein.

Even though scientific evidence to date is incomplete, it does suggest that antioxidant nutrients are part of a complex and interdependent defense system. As such, expecting any one of the elements in this system to operate effectively without the system synergy may be naïve at best. These nutrients seem to be more effective in concert with each other. This may be the underlying reason that fruits and vegetable intake always seems associated with health benefits, while consumption of selected components in the form of supplements does not always show efficacy. There will always be a debate regarding the benefits of deriving antioxidants from foods or supplements. In the final analysis food may be best for most people, but supplements necessary for some people under certain conditions. There is, however, a time element to these questions that are difficult for scientists to study. What are the effects of lifelong dietary habits versus lifelong supplement habits? Why do animals produce far more vitamin C themselves via biosynthesis than we can consume in food alone? There is much more basic science to be done.

RECOMMENDATIONS

All patients should be encouraged to improve their intake of antioxidant nutrients and phytochemicals through a plant-based diet. Until such time that scientific evidence makes a case for change, patients who are under oxidative stress due to illness or other causes and those wishing to supplement their diets should be advised not to exceed safe intake levels advised by the Food and Nutrition Board of the IOM. For use of any dietary supplement it is best to consult the Office of Dietary Supplements (ODS) fact sheets available on their Web site (see Appendix C).[163]

5

THE ANTIOXIDANTS OF LIFE

As we have seen, antioxidant studies in humans have produced conflicting results. While it is apparent they play a vital role in the biology of life, their ability to improve our health and prolong our life has yet to be proven beyond a shadow of a doubt. Health professionals have not reached a unified consensus about what to recommend to their patients, and public perceptions of antioxidants, while clearly more positive and trusting, pose serious safety concerns. What we do know is that there are many synergistic interactions between compounds within the food matrix, bodily enzymes and hormones, and antioxidants themselves. It may very well be these synergies that account for the health benefits we attribute to antioxidants alone.

There are a number of biological substances and compounds that exhibit antioxidant activity. Some are exogenous vitamins, some are endogenous enzymes, some are mineral cofactors, and some exert their effects by modulating endogenous oxidative defense mechanisms. Confusion about what represents a "true" antioxidant is exhibited by the case of the mineral selenium. Even though it is considered an "antioxidant," selenium is actually an essential dietary micronutrient that is incorporated into selenoproteins. Selenoproteins are proteins that exhibit antioxidant characteristics, thereby giving selenium antioxidant status. Antioxidants can be classified into two groups: endogenous and exogenous.

Endogenous Antioxidants	Exogenous Antioxidants
Superoxide dismutase	Vitamin C
Glutathione peroxidase	Vitamin E
Ubiquinone (Co-enzyme Q10)	Carotenoids
Thioredoxin reductase	Selenium
Catalase	Polyphenols

Like vitamins, they are either water soluble or fat soluble. The water-soluble antioxidants react with oxidants in cell cytoplasm and blood plasma. The fat-soluble antioxidants protect cell membranes from lipid peroxidation. Antioxidant interactions between each other, enzymes, or metabolites affect how they function in the human body and antioxidant protection depends upon synergies, body concentration, and reactivity with free radicals they encounter. We have looked at the endogenous antioxidant in a previous chapter and will now focus on the exogenous antioxidant for the remainder of this chapter.

VITAMIN A AND CAROTENOIDS

Carotenoids are the red, orange, and yellow pigments found in fruits and vegetables that give them their colorful appearance. There are more than 600 different forms of carotenoids and they are actually vitamin precursors, also known as provitamins. Vitamin A and carotenoids are closely connected. Many theories exist about the functions of carotenoids, but their only known function is conversion into vitamin A when vitamin A stores are low. Forms of vitamin A included retinol, retinal, retinoic acid, and retinyl esters. The most common carotenoids found in the North American diet are alpha-carotene (α-carotene), beta-carotene (β-carotene), beta-cryptoxanthin (β-cryptoxanthin), lycopene, lutein, and zeaxanthin. Only α-carotene, β-carotene, and β-cryptoxanthin can be converted by the body into preformed vitamin A retinol (although at a lower bioavailability than from animal sources) and are called provitamin A carotenoids. Lycopene, lutein, and zeaxanthin cannot be converted into vitamin A and are known as nonprovitamin A carotenoids.[1]

All carotenoids are fat-soluble and metabolized in the intestine. Therefore, a fat source must be included with them in a meal for the carotenoids to be absorbed. Eventually they are taken up by the liver and, if needed, converted to retinal (another form of vitamin A). Since vitamin A is fat-soluble and therefore stored by the body, carotenoids will be converted to vitamin A only if body stores of vitamin A are low.

Carotenoids, lycopene in particular, are considered antioxidants because they are effective at quenching singlet oxygen. It is theorized that carotenoids inhibit lipid peroxidation under some conditions, increase communication between cells, therefore lowering cancer risk, increase immune system function, have a role in cardiovascular disease prevention, and lower risk for macular degeneration and cataracts. But it is still unclear if these potential functions are the result of the actual carotenoid or due to synergistic interactions.

As we saw in previous chapters, study results in humans have been mixed. While some studies report carotenoid supplements are beneficial, two large studies—the CARET study and the ATBC Trial—actually found that death risk increased in some cases with carotenoid dietary supplementation.[2]

SAFETY ISSUES

Because carotenoids will convert into vitamin A only when body stores are low, they are only needed when vitamin A is consistently deficient in the diet. Vitamin A is needed for vision, growth, reproduction, and immunity. Requirements for vitamin A depend on how much is stored in the liver and absorption is affected by the amount of fat in the diet, the food matrix, food processing, and absence of intestinal infections. Hypervitaminosis A (excess intake of vitamin A) is toxic and can be acute or chronic. Acute toxicity usually occurs when retinol intake is over 150,000 μg in adults and 5,500 μg in infants. Chronic toxicity occurs when retinol intakes exceed 30,000 μg per day over a period of time in adults.[3] Specific population groups—those who abuse alcohol and/or those with liver disease, hyperlipidemia, or severe protein malnutrition—often have increased requirements for vitamin A over those in the general population.

Provitamin A carotenoids have no reported deficiencies (as long as vitamin A is adequately consumed) or toxicities. Likewise, non-provitamin A carotenoids have no reported toxicities or deficiencies. However, overconsumption of β-carotene (30 mg/day or more from supplements over long periods of time) can result in a non-life-threatening medical condition known as carotenodermia, which is a yellow discoloration of the skin. Likewise, excess lycopene intake (by overconsuming lycopene rich foods) can cause a deep orange skin discoloration known as lycopenodermia. These skin discolorations usually disappear once supplement intake is reduced or discontinued.

Special Considerations

Smokers, teenagers, young adults, and those who ingest excess alcohol have been found to have lower plasma levels of carotenoids. It is uncertain if this is due to age, lifestyle choice, or because fruit and vegetable intake is generally poor in these individuals. Supplementing these at risk groups with carotenoid supplements has been shown to be beneficial; however caution is advised with smokers. As the CARET and ATBC studies found, cancer deaths increased when β-carotene dietary supplements were given to smokers (although it is interesting to note that cancer deaths did not increase when they were supplemented with β-carotene from food sources rather than from supplements).

Mineral oil, cholesterol-reducing drugs (such as cholestyramine and colestipol), the obesity drug Orlistat, Colchicine (used for treatment of gout), and regular use of plant sterol- or stanol-containing margarines have been shown to reduce carotenoid absorption from food sources and supplements. There is some evidence that alcohol may also inhibit β-carotene conversion to retinol.

Supplement versus Food Source

All the carotenoids—α-carotene, β-carotene, β-cryptoxanthin, lycopene, lutein, and zeaxanthin—are available as dietary supplements over-the-counter. Bioavailability (how much of the nutrient is available from the source for absorption by the body) can be as much as 65–75 percent when they are formulated using an oil base solution. Bioavailability from carotenoid food sources, however, can sometimes be as low as 2 percent and depends upon other factors (such as cooking method). The best dietary sources of vitamin A come from retinol (preformed vitamin A) that is found in animal foods (such as liver, dairy products, and fish) and vitamin A fortified foods (such as grains, margarine, low- and nonfat milk). As noted before, vitamin A is also supplied by the provitamin A carotenoids (available in fruits and vegetables such as carrots, squash, peas, spinach, collard greens, cantaloupe, and broccoli). Cooking fruits and vegetables with 3–5 grams of fat (equivalent to one teaspoon of oil or margarine) increases the bioavailability of carotenoids from foods. Steaming also appears to be the best cooking method to maximize bioavailability, although overcooking will reduce available carotenoids.[4]

Individuals at risk of vitamin A deficiency (hospitalized children between six and twenty-four months, patients with gastrointestinal or pancreatic disorders, vegetarians, those with iron or zinc deficiencies, or patients with erythropoietic protoporphyria [extreme skin sensitivity to sunlight due to an enzyme deficiency and treated with β-carotene]) may benefit from carotenoid dietary supplements under medical supervision. Table 5.1 provides a listing of carotenoid and vitamin A food sources.[5]

RECOMMENDATIONS

Study results from the 1986 NHIS found that 26 percent of American adults took a vitamin A supplement. NHANES III, 1994–1996 data found the highest mean intake amount of preformed vitamin A for any gender and life stage group was between 895 and 1,503 μg/d, and, of those who took vitamin A supplements, approximately 1,500 to 3,000 μg/d was the maximum ingested. Therefore, the Food and Nutrition Board of the IOM of the National Academies concluded that the risk for exceeding the UL for vitamin A was small based on this data. Deficiency concerns were also felt to be minimal, except for those individuals within a subgroup of the population at risk for vitamin A deficiency. Based on all the evidence to date, the Food and Nutrition Board has concluded that while carotenoids appear beneficial and are vital for metabolism, more studies need to be evaluated and DRIs for carotenoids cannot be established at this time. At least five or more dietary servings of fruits and vegetables on a daily basis are recommended for the general population as the preferred source for both vitamin A and carotenoids. Caution is advised when using vitamin A or carotenoid supplements, especially for those with liver disease or alcohol abuse, hyperlipidemia, or severe protein malnutrition. While they show an increased need for them, these individuals also appear to have an increased susceptibility to excess preformed vitamin A and toxicities. Supplements should only be taken under medical supervision.[6] DRIs for vitamin A and carotenoids are provided in Appendix B.

Table 5.1
Common Vitamin A & Carotenoid Food Sources

Food Sources	Serving Size	α-Carotene (μg)	β-carotene (μg)	β-cryptoxanthin (μg)	Lycopene (μg)	Lutein & Zeaxanthin (μg)	Vitamin A (IU)*
Apricots							
juice	½ cup	–	–	–	–	–	2,063
nectar	½ cup	–	–	–	–	–	1,651
Baked beans, canned	1 cup	–	–	–	1,298	–	–
Broccoli, frozen, cooked	1 cup	–	–	–	–	2,756	–
Brussel sprouts, frozen, cooked	1 cup	–	–	–	–	2,389	–
Carrots							
raw	1 medium	2,028	–	–	–	–	8,666
cooked	1 cup	5,891	12,998	315	–	–	26,836
juice	8 ounces	10,247	21,955	–	–	–	45,134
Cantaloupe, raw	1 cup	–	3,232	–	–	–	5,411
Cheese, cheddar	1 ounce	–	–	–	–	–	284
Collards, frozen, cooked	1 cup	216	11,591	–	–	18,527	–
Corn, yellow, frozen, cooked	1 cup	–	–	200	–	1,586	–
Dandelion greens, cooked	1 cup	–	6,248	–	–	4,944	–
Egg							
raw, fresh, whole	1 large	–	–	–	–	–	244
cooked, hard boiled	1 large	–	–	–	–	–	293
Egg substitute	¼ cup						226
Grapefruit, pink, raw	½ grapefruit	–	–	–	1,745	–	–
Kale, frozen, cooked	1 cup	–	11,470	–	–	25,606	19,116
Liver							
beef, cooked	3 ounces	–	–	–	–	–	27,185
chicken, cooked	3 ounces	–	–	–	–	–	12,325

(continued)

Table 5.1 *(continued)*

Food Sources	Serving Size	α-Carotene (μg)	β-carotene (μg)	β-cryptoxanthin (μg)	Lycopene (μg)	Lutein & Zeaxanthin (μg)	Vitamin A (IU)*
Mango, sliced	1 cup	–	–	–	–	–	1,262
Milk							
fortified, skim	1 cup	–	–	–	–	–	500
fortified, whole	1 cup	–	–	–	–	–	249
Mixed vegetables, frozen, cooked	1 cup	1,762	–	–	–	–	–
Mustard greens, cooked	1 cup	–	–	–	–	8,347	–
Nectarines, raw	1 medium	–	–	133	–	–	–
Oatmeal, instant, fortified, plain	1 cup	–	–	–	–	–	1,252
Oranges							
raw	1 medium	–	–	152	–	–	–
juice, fresh	8 ounces	–	–	419	–	–	–
Papaya, raw	1 cup	–	–	2,313	–	–	1,532
Paprika, dried	1 tsp.	–	–	166	–	–	–
Peaches							
raw	1 medium	–	–	–	–	–	319
canned	1/2 cup	85	–	–	–	–	473
Peas, frozen, cooked	1 cup	784	–	–	–	3,840	2,100
Plantains, raw	1 medium	–	–	–	–	–	–
Peppers							
red, sweet, cooked	1 cup	–	–	2,817	–	–	–
raw	1 medium	–	–	583	459	–	313
Pumpkin							
canned	1 cup	11,748	17,003	–	–	–	–
pie	1 piece	748	7,366	–	–	–	–
cooked	1 cup	–	–	3,553	–	2,484	–

Soup, vegetable, canned	1 cup	—	—	—	—	—	5,820
Spinach							
frozen, cooked	1 cup	—	13,750	—	—	29,811	22,916
raw	1 cup	—	—	—	—	—	2,813
Squash							
summer, cooked	1 cup	1,398	5,726	—	—	4,048	—
winter, baked	1 cup	—	—	—	—	2,901	—
Sweet Potato, baked	1 medium	—	16,803	—	—	—	—
Tangerines, raw	1 medium	85	—	342	—	—	—
Tomatoes							
raw	1 medium	124	—	—	4,631	—	—
paste, canned	1 cup	—	—	—	75,362	—	—
puree, canned	1 cup	—	—	—	54,385	—	—
marinara sauce	1 cup	—	—	—	39,975	—	—
juice, canned	8 ounces	—	—	—	21,960	—	1,092
soup	1 cup	—	—	—	25,615	—	—
catsup	1 Tbsp.	—	—	—	2,551	—	—
Turnip greens, frozen, cooked	1 cup	—	10,593	—	—	19,541	—
Vegetable Juice, canned	8 ounces	—	—	—	23,337	—	—
Watermelon, raw	1 wedge	—	—	223	12,962	—	—

*1 IU=0.3 µg retinol

Source: Adapted from Higdon, "Dietary Supplement Fact Sheet: Vitamin A and Carotenoids," The Linus Pauling Institute (2005) and Office of Dietary Supplements, 2005.

VITAMIN C

As discussed previously, vitamin C or ascorbic acid is an essential water-soluble vitamin for all humans and functions as an antioxidant and cofactor in enzyme and hormonal reactions. It has been promoted as increasing immunity, thereby preventing and reducing colds. However, studies have yet to support this long-standing theory. It does play a major role in cartilage and collagen formation, in regulation of iron absorption and storage, and in immune system protection. Vitamin C scavenges free radicals (by donating electrons) and re-generates other biological antioxidants (such as glutathione and α-tocopherol [vitamin E]). The body does not store vitamin C because it is water-soluble, although the body does have small tissue storage pools up to 2,000 mg. Excess intake is excreted and, in times of low dietary intake, the body will conserve vitamin C by minimizing excretion.[7]

Vitamin C supplementation has been associated with lowered risk for cardiovascular diseases (especially in diabetics), some cancers, cataracts, and lead toxicity. Most studies show mixed results, but there have been some promising findings. Vitamin C appears to reduce gastric cancers by eradicating *helicobacter pylori* (*H. pylori*—a bacteria associated with increased stomach cancers), stomach ulcers, and lower vitamin C concentrations in gastric secretions. Lower blood lead levels have also been observed when vitamin C supplements are taken. Both positive and negative outcomes have been observed in diabetics with cardiovascular disease and genetic factors appear to play more of an important role in how effective vitamin C supplements are in diabetics.

While vitamin C has proven itself to be a very effective antioxidant in the lab, how well it functions in the human body remains to be seen. It should be mentioned that some studies have found vitamin C can turn into a pro-oxidant, causing cell damage due to production of oxygen byproducts. However, these studies are felt to have flawed study designs and shed doubt upon their findings.[8]

SAFETY ISSUES

Vitamin C is absorbed through the intestine and is regulated by the kidney. In general, no toxicities have been observed with high doses. But doses over 3,000 mg per day[9] have been associated with gastrointestinal disturbances, such as diarrhea, nausea, and abdominal cramping. Other adverse effects such as kidney stone formation, "rebound scurvy" (where symptoms of scurvy develop because the body adapts to high levels of vitamin C and then becomes "deficient" when intakes are decreased back to normal levels), increased iron absorption leading to hemochromatosis (iron overload), reduced vitamin B_{12} and copper tissue absorption levels, increased oxygen demand, and erosion of dental enamel have been experienced but none confirmed. Symptoms associated with high intakes often resolve once intake is reduced or discontinued. Because the body can experience adverse effects from large doses, the Food and Nutrition Board for the first time in DRI history recommended a UL for vitamin C.

Vitamin C deficiencies are rare in most industrialized countries. Deficiencies are occasionally seen among individuals with poor fruit and vegetable intake or excess drug and alcohol use. As we saw in a previous chapter, the classic vitamin C deficiency disease is scurvy. Symptoms of scurvy include inflamed and bleeding gums, impaired wound healing, joint pain, joint effusion (escape of fluid from the joints), hyperkeratosis (thickening of the outer layer of skin), petechiae (hemorrhaging of blood vessels in the skin), and ecchymoses (skin discoloration caused by bruising). Shortness of breath, edema, dry eyes and mouth, weakness, fatigue, and depression have also been associated with vitamin C deficiency.

SPECIAL CONSIDERATIONS

In the United States, smokers and passive smokers, men (particularly the elderly), those in lower socioeconomic classes, those with poor fruit and vegetable intake, drug and alcohol abusers, and those with chronic diseases and disabilities (particularly hemochromatosis and renal disease) are at a higher risk for low blood levels of vitamin C. Some pharmaceutical drugs—birth control pills and aspirin (when taken frequently)—are known to lower vitamin C levels in the body as well. There is some evidence that vitamin C can interact with anticoagulant medications (such as coumadin) and high doses have been found to affect lab test results. Therefore, it is extremely important for patients to report vitamin C supplement use to their health care providers and to discontinue use of vitamin C dietary supplements at least two weeks prior to any planned blood or urine testing.

SUPPLEMENT VERSUS FOOD SOURCE

Fruits and vegetables are the primary food sources for vitamin C. Citrus fruits and juices, tomatoes, tomato products, tomato juice, and potatoes are the most popular sources in the American diet. But vitamin C is also found in brussel sprouts, cauliflower, broccoli, strawberries, cabbage, spinach, and foods fortified with vitamin C. Time and condition of the growing season, growing location, cooking practices, and storage time before consumption can all affect the amount of vitamin C available from a food source. Table 5.2 lists common vitamin C dietary sources.[10] Vitamin C bioavailability from food sources and dietary supplements appears to be similar and both have an estimated 70 to 90 percent absorption rate by the body. As expected, absorption rates do decrease when intake increases beyond physiological needs.[11]

RECOMMENDATIONS

Data from the NHANES III, 1988–1994 found the highest mean intakes of vitamin C from both diet and supplements for all gender and life stage

Table 5.2
Common Vitamin C Food Sources

Food Source	Serving Size	Vitamin C (mg)
Broccoli, cooked	$^1/_2$ cup	58
Brussel sprouts, cooked	$^1/_2$ cup	48
Cabbage, cooked	$^1/_2$ cup	15
Cauliflower, cooked	$^1/_2$ cup	27
Grapefruit		
fresh	$^1/_2$ medium	44
juice	6 ounces	60
Orange		
fresh	1 medium	70
juice	6 ounces	75
Pepper, sweet, red, raw	$^1/_2$ cup	141
Potato		
baked	1 medium	26
sweet, baked	1 medium	22
Spinach		
frozen, cooked	$^1/_2$ cup	2
raw	$^1/_2$ cup	4
Strawberries, fresh, whole	1 cup	82
Tomato		
fresh	1 medium	23
juice	1 cup	45
sauce	1 cup	32

Source: Adapted from Higdon, "Vitamin C," The Linus Pauling Institute, 2006.

groups was about 200 mg/d, with 1,200mg/d the highest reported intake.[12] The Food and Nutrition Board concluded that Americans are unlikely to exceed the UL for vitamin C from both food and supplements. They also determined that supplementing the American diet with vitamin C does not appear to result in added health benefits. Therefore the Food and Nutrition Board recommends intake of vitamin C should come from at least five servings of fruits and vegetables daily. Those population groups at risk for vitamin C deficiency (poor fruit and vegetable intakes or those with oxidative stresses [smokers, nonsmokers, alcohol and drug abusers]) may benefit from added vitamin C dietary supplements under medical supervision. Those using anti-coagulant medications should avoid dietary supplements, unless otherwise directed by their physician. DRI recommendations for vitamin C are provided in Appendix B.

VITAMIN E

Vitamin E is an essential fat-soluble nutrient. There are eight compounds, called tocols, which exhibit vitamin E activity. But only one, alpha-tocopherol (α-tocopherol), is considered the biologically active form used by humans. Vitamin E strengthens red blood cell membranes, acts as a chain-breaking antioxidant preventing the spread of free radical reactions, synthesizes heme (the deep red portion of hemoglobin that contains iron in red blood cells) and essential body compounds, and supports cellular respiration. It is also thought to improve vasodilation and inhibit platelets from clumping together in the bloodstream. While vitamin E is absorbed in the intestine, it is the liver that actually differentiates between the different tocols, taking up α-tocopherol and secreting it in very low density lipoproteins (LDLs).

SAFETY ISSUES

In the United States vitamin E deficiencies are rare. When they do occur it is usually due to genetic abnormalities of α-tocopherol metabolism, fat malabsorption diseases (such as Crohn's disease or cystic fibrosis), prematurity of infants, protein-energy malnutrition, or zinc deficiency. Symptoms of vitamin E deficiency include peripheral neuropathy, muscle weakness and ataxia, retinopathy, and red blood cell anemia. A 2005 MSNBC article noted that about 93 percent of Americans fail to consume recommended levels of vitamin E (based on NHANES data) mainly due to dieting efforts that cut back on calories and reduce fat intake.[13] The IOM findings differ with this conclusion and the Food and Nutrition Board concludes vitamin E consumption to be adequate overall. However, individuals who eat low-fat and/or low-calorie diets may be at risk for low intakes of vitamin E and possible deficiencies.

There are no reported adverse effects from excess consumption of vitamin E from foods. However, toxicity from long-term excess vitamin E dietary supplements, which are in both natural and synthetic forms of tocopherols, is still unknown. A tendency to hemorrhage can occur if supplement doses exceed 1,500 IU (1000 mg) of natural α-tocopherol or 1,100 IU of synthetic and is the basis for establishing an UL for vitamin E.[14]

SPECIAL CONSIDERATIONS

Premature infants are at risk for hemolytic anemia due to vitamin E deficiency. However, they are also very susceptible to toxic effects of α-tocopherol supplementation and vitamin E must be carefully used and monitored with them. Patients who are deficient in vitamin K or on anticoagulant therapy may also experience hemorrhagic toxicity and decreased blood coagulation if taking excess vitamin E doses. A 2005 study reported in the *Journal of the National Cancer Institute* found that head and neck cancer patients were at risk for recurrence of their cancers and at a greater risk for developing a second primary cancer when taking 400 IU of α-tocopherol supplements during and after radiation therapy.[15] Therefore, cancer patients would be wise to avoid dietary vitamin E supplementation.

SUPPLEMENT VERSUS FOOD SOURCE

Dietary sources of vitamin E are vegetable oils (sunflower, cottonseed, safflower, canola, olive, palm, rice-bran, and wheat-germ oils), unprocessed cereal grains, nuts, fruits, and vegetables. Food sources contain both α-tocopherol and gamma-tocopherol (γ-tocopherol). While γ-tocopherol is more abundant in foods and exhibits antioxidant activity, its function and absorption is still relatively unknown. Table 5.3 provides a list of common vitamin E dietary sources.[16]

There are both natural and synthetic formulations of vitamin E supplements in the market. Natural vitamin E supplements usually contain the α-tocopherol form of vitamin E, while the synthetic formulations contain mixed tocopherols (although some natural do contain mixed tocopherols as well). As a rule, it has been found that natural forms of α-tocopherol are better absorbed by the body than synthetic forms. Bioavailability appears to be the same from both dietary supplements and food sources. Although vitamin E absorption is also enhanced when a fat source is added to a meal, it must be remembered that most food sources of vitamin E already include fat and adding fat to the diet is a more important consideration when taking vitamin E dietary supplements or when a low-fat diet is followed.

Table 5.3
Common Vitamin E Food Sources

Food Sources
Almonds, dry roasted
Avocado
Broccoli, frozen, boiled
Cereal, fortified
Hazelnuts, dry roasted
Mango, raw
Mayonnaise
Oil
corn
soybean
safflower
sunflower
wheat
germ
Peanuts, dry roasted
Peanut butter, smooth
Spinach—raw, frozen, boiled
Sunflower seed kernels
Tomato, paste, canned, marinara sauce
Wheat germ

Source: Adapted from Hennekens et al., "Vitamin E," Office of Dietary Supplements, 2007.

Dietary nutrient databases and DRIs often report vitamin E in milligrams of α-tocopherol, while dietary supplement labels report vitamin E in IUs (international units). To determine how much α-tocopherol is provided by a dietary supplement, a conversion formula is used. Natural vitamin E dietary supplements use a conversion factor of 0.67. Synthetic formulations, as well as fortified foods and multivitamins, use a conversion factor of 0.45 because absorption rates are lower. For example, to calculate the α-tocopherol content of a natural vitamin E supplement containing 400 IU, multiply 400 IU by 0.67 to conclude that it contains 268 mg of α-tocopherol (400 ∗ 0.67 = 268).[17] A vitamin E conversion calculator is also available on the Internet and the URL is listed in Appendix C.

RECOMMENDATIONS

Data from the NHANES III, 1988–1994 found the highest mean intake of vitamin E from food and supplement sources for all genders and life stage groups was approximately 45 mg/d of α-tocopherol equivalents and a maximum reported intake of 508 mg/d. The Food and Nutrition Board concluded that use of vitamin E supplements in the United States was high based on data from the 1986 National Health Interview Survey (NHIS) (23 percent of men, 29 percent of women, and 37 percent of young children took a supplement that included vitamin E) and the Boston Nutritional Status Survey (1981–1984) (38 percent of men and 49 percent of women over the age of 60 took a vitamin E supplement containing vitamin E).[18]

The Food and Nutrition Board determined that the risk of excess intakes of vitamin E is very low. But because effects of long-term vitamin E supplementation are still unknown and hemorrhagic events have been observed with high doses of vitamin E intake, they recommend that vitamin E intake should come from food sources rather than dietary supplements. DRIs for vitamin E are provided in Appendix B. Premature infants and those with fat malabsorption or certain genetic diseases (such as abetalipoproteinemia, a rare disorder that interferes with fat and fat-soluble vitamin absorption) may need more vitamin E than the general population. Caution is also advised with premature infants, those with vitamin K deficiencies and on anticoagulant therapies, and those who follow low-fat diets.

SELENIUM

Selenium is a micronutrient used to defend against oxidative stresses, thus earning it antioxidant status. In reality, it is the selenoproteins (enzymes that include a selenocysteine residue) that exhibit the antioxidant activity that has captured attention. Selenium is important because it is an essential component of these selenoproteins. Selenoproteins are found in all living organisms and are ancient and well-conserved enzymes. However, while common in animals, they are rare or absent in algae, plants, and fungi. Selenium is a vital nutrient in animals and humans. A couple of dozen different selenocysteine-containing selenoproteins have been observed in human cells. Three selenoproteins—thioredoxin reductases 1 and 3 and glutathione peroxidase—have been shown to be essential. These enzymes are critical to endogenous oxidative defense systems and this is why selenium has been deemed essential to combat oxidative stress.

In addition to participating in antioxidant defense mechanisms, selenoproteins function in the regulation of thyroid hormone metabolism and the immune system. Excess selenium in the diet can cause toxic effects and result in selenium poisoning. Selenium deficiency limits the individual cell's ability to synthesize selenoproteins, and interruption of their synthesis is fatal to embryos. Thus, selenium is unique among all the minerals because small amounts in the diet can lead to deficiency symptoms and large amounts can become toxic or possibly carcinogenic. Selenium is used along with dietary protein to treat kwashiorkor, a form of malnutrition in children, and also has a protective effect on red blood cells and against mercury and cadmium toxicities. Research has found selenium may play a role in cancer, heart disease, arthritis, and HIV/AIDS. But study results are still inconclusive.

The glutathione peroxidases, including GPx1, GPx2, GPx3, and GPx4, are functionally the most important of all the selenoproteins. Three selenoproteins, which are iodothyronine deiodinases, regulate thyroid metabolism. Thioredoxin reductases regenerate vitamin C from oxidized metabolites and selenophosphate synthetase is involved in selenium metabolism. Selenide is the reduced form of selenium and all forms of selenium are eventually metabolized to this form.

Selenomethionine and selenocysteine are the two forms of selenium found in body tissues and in most dietary sources. Selenomethionine, synthesized by plants but not humans, is incorporated into dietary plant and animal proteins. Selenocysteine is found in animal selenoproteins and is the form used by humans in cell metabolism. Both forms are well absorbed by the body. Selenate and selenite are also found, but are not common in foods and are the forms usually added to functional foods/nutraceuticals and dietary supplements.

SAFETY ISSUES

Selenium can be toxic if consumed in large quantities because it closely resembles the mineral sulfur and can replace it in biochemical reactions while also inhibiting the action of some enzymes. However toxicity from inorganic selenium forms, found in dietary supplements and in occupations exposed to selenium dusts, is more likely to occur than from food sources. High-protein diets can reduce selenium toxicity risks. Symptoms of toxicity, which occur when selenium intakes from food, water, and supplement sources exceed 45–400 μg/d depending on age (see Appendix B), are irritability, nervous system abnormalities, hair and nail brittleness, gastrointestinal disturbances, fatigue, garlic breath odor, discolored or decayed teeth, and skin rashes or eruptions.

Selenium deficiency does not usually result in overt symptoms in well-nourished individuals. But it can predispose some to stress-related illnesses, such as Keshan and Kashin-Beck disease. Keshan disease occurs in selenium-deficient children under stress (such as an infection) and causes cardiomy-opathy. Kashin-Beck disease occurs in preadolescents or adolescents living in low-selenium farm areas and is an endemic disease of the cartilage.

SPECIAL CONSIDERATIONS

Selenium content of plant sources is dependent on the availability of selenium in the soil in which they are grown. While plants may vary in selenium content, muscle meats, milk, and eggs are more reliable food sources because selenium is added to animal feed in the United States and Canada. Western South Dakota and eastern Wyoming are designated by the USDA as areas for raising food animals only because they are high-selenium farming regions. Likewise, there are also low-selenium regions, but it is felt that the food-distribution system in the United States transports foods from such large and varied farm areas that a mix of both low- and high-selenium foods balances out these variations (although plant selenium content may vary considerably). Therefore, vegetarians and those who live in low-selenium farming regions may be at risk for low selenium intakes.

SUPPLEMENT VERSUS FOOD SOURCE

Food sources of selenium are meat, seafood, cereals and grains, dairy products, and fruits and vegetables. Drinking water has not been found to provide significant amounts of selenium in the diet. Table 5.4 provides a list of common selenium dietary sources.[19] Selenium from natural food sources has a higher bioavailability than functional foods/nutraceuticals and dietary supplements.

RECOMMENDATIONS

The Food and Nutrition Board concluded that foods are the best source of selenium intake. NHANES III, 1988–1994 data found the highest median intakes of selenium to be approximately 106 μg/d from food sources and 108 μg/d from supplements.[20] The 1986 NHIS found approximately 9 percent of Americans took dietary supplements containing selenium.[21] They concluded that the risk of exceeding the UL for selenium is low and that the general population meets its daily needs. Vegetarians and/or those living in low-selenium farming regions should choose foods carefully and may benefit

Table 5.4
Common Selenium Food Sources

Food Source	Serving Size	Selenium (μg)
Beef chuck roast, roasted	3 onces	23
Beef, cooked	$3\frac{1}{2}$ ounces	35
Brazil nuts, dried, unblanched	1 ounce	544*
Bread, enriched, wheat	1 slice	10
Bread, enriched, white	1 slice	4
Cheese, cheddar	1 ounce	4
Chicken breast, roasted	$3\frac{1}{2}$ ounces	20
Cod, cooked	3 ounces	32
Cottage Cheese, 2% fat	$\frac{1}{2}$ cup	12
Egg, whole, hard boiled	1 large	15
Macaroni, elbow, boiled	$\frac{1}{2}$ cup	15
Noodles, enriched, boiled	$\frac{1}{2}$ cup	17
Oatmeal, fort, instant, ckd	1 cup	12
Rice, brown, cooked	$\frac{1}{2}$ cup	10
Rice, white, cooked	$\frac{1}{2}$ cup	12
Spaghetti w/meat sauce	1 serving	34
Tuna, light, in oil	3 ounces	63
Turkey, light meat, roasted	$3\frac{1}{2}$ ounces	32
Walnuts, black, dried	1 ounce	5

Note: *Exceeds UL for selenium; quantities should be eaten in moderation.
Source: Adapted from Fahey et al., "Dietary Fact Sheet: Selenium," Office of Dietary Supplements, 2004.

from a multivitamin containing selenium. DRIs for selenium are provided in Appendix B.

POLYPHENOLS

Polyphenols are compounds found in plants that exhibit antioxidant activity and are theorized to reduce risk of cancers by blocking the action of enzymes and deactivating substances associated with cancer growth, reduce cardiovascular disease risk, and bind nonheme iron from plant sources thus decreasing absorption by the body. They include tannins, lignins, anthocyanins, catechins, epicatechin, stilbenes gallic acid, and flavonoids. In recent years, polyphenols have received almost daily media attention because of antioxidant, antiaging, and antiinflammatory properties that appear to protect cells from free radical damage.

Polyphenols, including the flavonoids, are ubiquitous in plant materials and especially so in foods, such as berries, tea, beer, wine, olive oil, chocolate and cocoa, walnuts, peanuts, fruit and fruit skins, and vegetables. Green tea has become popular in recent years because of the polyphenol epigallocatechin-3-gallate (EGCG), which has been shown in the lab to scavenge ROS and RNS.

The end result is protection of the fatty membranes of cells, proteins, and DNA thus preventing cancers. Some animal studies also show reduced rates of dementia with delayed loss of cognition and some restoration of function with aging.

Over 6,000 flavonoids have been identified in foods from plant sources.[22] It is theorized they reduce cardiovascular disease and cancer risk, but exactly which flavanoids are more protective under certain conditions remains to be more fully explored. Like all antioxidants, flavonoids also have the potential to turn into pro-oxidants once they have been oxidized. Chemically, reduction potentials of flavonoid radicals in neutral media are higher than that of vitamin C. Consequently, flavonoid radicals have the potential to oxidize and deplete vitamin C *in vivo*, although this has not yet been demonstrated. Some flavonoids such as epigallocatechin, epigallocatechin gallate, and quercetin are situated in the redox pecking order such that they could potentially repair the vitamin E radical and recycle vitamin E, but again this still has not yet been shown *in vivo*.

In general, flavonoids have poor absorption rates with rapid metabolism and excretion, limiting their ability to act as an antioxidant. Flavonoids also inhibit vitamin C transport into cells and can bind nonheme iron.

The polyphenolic flavonoids found in red wine and cocoa have received the most press attention. Red wine polyphenols are related to what is known as the "French Paradox," the term given to the observation that French people remain slim and have low incidences of coronary heart disease despite eating a diet high in saturated fats. It has been suggested that the tendency of the French to consume higher quantities of red wine (containing the polyphenol resveratrol) than Americans is the reason for lower heart disease rates. Study of the average French diet finds that portion sizes are smaller, dietary fats mostly come from dairy and vegetable sources (very little from animal fat), fish is eaten more often, snacking between meals is limited, convenience foods are avoided, and sugar intake is lower than the average American diet. It is most likely these reasons, and not resveratrol, that account for the difference in cardiovascular disease rates between the two countries.

Cocoa polyphenols have also received quite a bit of attention because many Americans love chocolate. Large candy makers—Nestle' and Mars in particular—have invested large sums in cocoa research and new product development in the hopes of benefiting financially from the current antioxidant "craze." But as with red wine, science has yet to prove cocoa polyphenol benefits.

Research into the benefits of polyphenols is still in the infancy stages. No definite benefits or adverse events have been seen to date and there are no DRIs for polyphenolic compounds currently. As with all other antioxidants, it is recommended that an increased and varied diet of fruits and vegetables (between five to nine servings daily), legumes, and whole grains is beneficial. Table 5.5 lists common dietary polyphenol sources.[23]

Table 5.5
Common Polyphenols

Dietary Polyphenols	Common Food Sources
Anthocyanidins	Berries—red, blue, & purple Cherries Grapes—red & purple Plums Red wine Rhubarb
Flavanols	Apples Berries Chocolate Grapes—green & red Red wine Teas—green, white, black, oolong
Flavanones	Citrus fruits & juice—orange, grapefruit, lemon
Flavonols	Apples Berries Broccoli Kale Scallions Teas Yellow onions
Flavones	Celery Hot peppers Parsley Thyme
Isoflavones	Legumes Soy foods Soybeans
Catechin, Epicatechin	Apples, cider Apricots Beans Blackberries Cherries Grapes Peaches Red wine Teas—black & green
Hydroxybenzoic acids (gallic)	Black currant Blackberries Raspberries Strawberries

Table 5.5 *(continued)*

Dietary Polyphenols	Common Food Sources
Proanthocyanidins	Apples
	Apricots
	Avocados
	Bananas
	Beans—red kidney, pinto, black
	Beer
	Berries
	Cherries
	Chocolate
	Cinnamon
	Curry
	Grapes—green, grape seed
	Indian squash
	Juices—cranberry, apple, grape
	Kiwis
	Mangos
	Nectarines
	Nuts
	Peaches
	Pears
	Plums
	Red wine

Source: Adapted from Buhler and Miranda,"Antioxidant Activities of Flavonoids," The Linus Pauling Institute, 2000; Manach et al., "Polyphenols: Food Sources and Bioavailability," *The Am J Clin Nutr* 79 (2004): 727–747.

ZINC AND COENZYME Q10

Zinc and coenzyme Q10 (CoQ10) are compounds that need to be mentioned because they appear to have a close connection to antioxidant activity. Zinc, an essential micronutrient, is found in almost every cell and serves as a catalyst for enzymes, supports a healthy immune system, aids wound healing, is required in DNA synthesis, is required for growth and development during pregnancy, childhood, and adolescence, and maintains the senses of taste and smell. It is found in a wide variety of foods, but good sources are oysters, red meat, poultry, some shellfish, beans, nuts, whole grains, fortified breakfast cereals, and dairy products. Bioavailability is greater from animal sources than plant sources. Phytates (plant phosphorus that binds minerals making them unavailable for absorption) in plant sources (whole grains, cereal, and legumes) can bind zinc, thus decreasing its bioavailability. Zinc absorption can also be inhibited by iron, calcium, phosphorus, protein, fiber, and picolinate (a metal salt used as an intermediate in dietary supplements). Table 5.6 provides a listing of common zinc food sources.[24]

Table 5.6
Common Zinc Food Sources

Food Source	Serving Size	Zinc (mg)
Almonds, dry roasted	1 ounce	1.0
Baked beans		
plain, canned	$^1/_2$ cup	1.7
with pork, canned	$^1/_2$ cup	1.8
Beef (pot roast, tenderloin, eye round, lean)	3 ounces	4.9
Cashews, dry roasted	1 ounce	1.6
Cheese		
swiss	1 ounce	1.1
cheddar	1 ounce	0.9
mozzarella, skim	1 ounce	0.9
Chicken		
breast (no skin, no bone)	$^1/_2$ ounces	1
leg	1 leg	2.7
Chickpeas, canned	$^3/_4$ cup	1.3
Flounder/sole, cooked	3 ounces	0.5
Kidney beans, cooked	$^1/_2$ cup	0.8
Milk, any kind	1 cup	0.9
Mixed nuts, dry roasted	1 ounce	1.1
Oatmeal, instant	1 package	0.8
Oysters, battered, fried	6 medium	16
Peas, frozen, boiled	$^1/_2$ cup	0.8
Pecans, dry roasted	1 ounce	1.4
Pork loins	3 ounces	2.4
Ready-to-eat cereals (fortified with zinc)	$^3/_4$ cup	1.5
Raisin Bran	$^3/_4$ cup	1.3
Walnuts, black, dried	1 ounce	1.0
Wheat Bran flakes	$^3/_4$ cup	3.7
Yogurt		
plain, low fat	1 cup	2.2
fruit, low fat	1 cup	1.6

Source: Adapted from "Facts about Dietary Supplements: Zinc," Office of Dietary Supplements, 2002.

NHANES III, 1988–1994 data found the highest median zinc intakes from food and supplements was 25–32 mg/d for adult men and nonpregnant adult women and 40–47 mg/d for pregnant and lactating women. Approximately 24 mg/d for adult men was ingested from food sources only.[25] Zinc deficiencies are rare and those with malabsorption diseases (celiac sprue, Crohn's disease, and short bowel syndrome) or who have a low caloric intake, impaired growth, or excess alcohol intake are at risk for deficiency. Deficiency symptoms include hair loss, diarrhea, growth retardation, delayed sexual maturation and impotence, eye and skin lesions, and loss of appetite. The genetic disease acrodermatitis enteropathica is a zinc malabsorption disease and causes severe skin lesions and cognitive dysfunction.

There is no evidence of zinc toxicity from excess intake from food sources. However, adverse effects can occur when intakes between 50 and 450 mg of supplemental zinc are taken.[26] Symptoms include suppression of the immune system, epigastric pain, nausea, vomiting, loss of appetite, headaches, diarrhea, cramps, decreased high density lipoproteins (HDL), and reduced copper, folate, and iron absorption. Those with Menke's disease (a genetic disease affecting copper metabolism that primarily affects infants) may be susceptible to the effects of excess zinc intake as well.

Coenzyme Q10 (CoQ10), a ubiquinone, is found in cell mitochondria. It is a fat-soluble compound synthesized by the body and also found in foods. A vitamin-like compound, it is used as a coenzyme in cell energy production and theorized to scavenge free radicals and improve heart function. CoQ10 is found in meat, poultry, fish, soybean and canola oils, sardines, mackerel, fruits, vegetables, eggs, dairy products, and nuts. Frying vegetables and eggs can decrease their CoQ10 bioavailability between 14 to 32 percent, but boiling does not change bioavailability. Table 5.7 lists common CoQ10 food sources.[27]

There are no known toxicities from CoQ10 dietary supplements, but some people have reported nausea, diarrhea, appetite suppression, heartburn, and abdominal discomfort with excess intake. Interactions with statin drugs and anticoagulants have also been reported and CoQ10 supplements should be avoided when these medications are taken. No deficiencies have been reported

Table 5.7
Common CoQ10 Food Sources

Food Source	Serving Size	CoQ10 (mg)
Beef, fried	3 ounces	2.6
Broccoli, boiled	1/2 cup	0.5
Cauliflower, boiled	1/2 cup	0.4
Chicken, fried	3 ounces	1.4
Egg, boiled	1 medium	0.1
Herring, marinated	3 ounces	2.3
Oil		
soybean	1 Tbsp.	1.3
canola	1 Tbsp.	1.0
Orange	1 medium	0.3
Peanuts, roasted	1 ounce	0.8
Pistachio nuts, roasted	1 ounce	0.6
Sesame seeds, roasted	1 ounce	0.7
Strawberries	1/2 cup	0.1
Trout, rainbow, steamed	3 ounces	0.9

Source: Adapted from Higdon, "Coenzyme Q10," The Linus Pauling Institute, 2007.

and it is assumed that normal biosynthesis and a varied diet meet daily needs for healthy individuals. CoQ10 supplements do appear to benefit individuals with rare mitochondrial diseases, such as mitochondrial encephalomyopathies. At this time there are no DRI recommendations for CoQ10.

As we can see, more studies need to be done on the antioxidants of life to truly determine just what their exact role in health and aging is and how effective they really are. Caution is highly advised when taking any of them in supplement form and should only be done so with medical advice. The evidence to date supports incorporating a variety of foods—most notably fruits, vegetables, legumes, and whole grains—into the daily diet as the best way to achieve adequate intakes of antioxidants and positively influence health outcomes.

6

MAKING SENSE OF IT ALL

As research studies till date show, consistent evidence supporting antioxidant benefits in human trials has been disappointing. In vitro and animal studies suggest antioxidant supplementation provides benefits, however, some recent research demonstrates that in some cases antioxidant supplementation may actually do more harm than good. Individual antioxidants in the form of dietary supplements are more potent and bioavailable than they are in food matrices, and they do not exhibit the synergistic effects with other compounds found within natural food sources. Therefore, supplements most likely do not possess all the physiologically active components needed to be truly effective in preventing disease incidence and progression. In addition, individual genetics and/or physical status may have as significant an effect on health as antioxidant nutrients do. We saw in the early years of America that poor diets caused many nutrition-related, life-threatening, and debilitating diseases. Food fortification programs, such as vitamin D and iodine, proved to be beneficial and improved public health by eradicating or preventing most associated illnesses. Today nutrition deficiencies are rare in America. Poor diet is usually the result of individual choice, lack of knowledge, extreme poverty, or illness. The average American has the opportunity to obtain his or her daily nutrient needs from diet alone. Nevertheless, many Americans do not achieve optimal levels of vitamin C and E and perhaps the flavonoids.

There are also some suspicions that the food supply (specifically fruits and vegetables) is not as nutritious as it once was. At least one study carried out at the University of Texas at Austin found six out of thirteen major nutrients in fruits and vegetables (protein, calcium, phosphorus, iron, riboflavin, and ascorbic acid) have declined over the past few decades (see Table 6.1). Analyzing these studies is difficult as they depend upon analytical techniques that vary over the decades. Nevertheless, it is reasonable to assume that farming practices that increase crop yields (and profits) over time may deplete natural resource capabilities and result in what is known as the "dilution effect" when crops are grown in the same locations for a number of years. This dilution of

Table 6.1
Changes in Nutrient Content of USDA Crops

Nutrient	Decrease in Nutrition Value (1950–1999)
Protein	6%
Calcium	16%
Phosphorus	9%
Iron	15%
Riboflavin	38%
Ascorbic acid (vitamin C)	20%

Source: Adapted from Davis, "Changes in USDA Food Composition Data for 43 Garden Crops, 1950 to 1999," *J of Am Coll of Nutr* 23, no. 6 (2004): 669–682.

minerals and vitamins in fruit and vegetable crops is the consequence of higher crop yields and shortened growing time (slower-growing crops have more time to absorb nutrients from the soil and sun).[1] Some studies of organic crops have shown increased nutrient values over conventional crops. A review of studies reported in *The Journal of Alternative and Complementary Medicine* in 2001 found vitamin C, iron, magnesium, and phosphorus values were significantly increased (along with decreased nitrates from fertilizers) when compared to conventionally grown crops. Yet, even this field of study yields conflicting results.[2] The theory that organic crops must combat more stresses as they grow, due to less protection from pesticides, appears to increase their nutrient and antioxidant phenolic values.[3] But these study results have yet to be verified over the long term.

Possible decreased nutrient value of crops and an aging population that is living longer, has more disposable income, believes supplements to be safe and effective, and is willing to self-medicate in an effort to feel better and decrease health care costs has driven the popularity and increased use of antioxidant supplement sales. Almost daily media reports extolling the virtues of antioxidants for increased longevity and improved health have steadily increased this trend in use of antioxidant dietary supplements and functional foods/nutraceuticals. Some companies allow consumers to "custom design" their nutrients by offering single portion packets of nutrients, such as a mix of vitamin C and iron that can be sprinkled onto foods.[4] Companies such as Pharmanex offer to a vulnerable public the BipPhotonic Scanner, which scans the skin on the palm of the hand for body carotenoid levels, and antioxidant testing kits (for $60 a urine sample) for testing oxidative stress levels. However, this scan measures only carotenoids and is not a true reflection of actual antioxidant levels in the body. Regarding the urine tests currently available, Garry Handelman, a nutrition professor at the University of Massachusetts, sums it up best: "I won't say that they're completely worthless, but they're about as close as they can get."[5]

Years of self-promoting lobbying efforts by the dietary supplement industry that urged Congress to preserve consumer freedom of choice and Congress, believing that all supplements were safe, allowed passage of DSHEA in 1994.[6] DSHEA effectively deregulated supplements and weakened the FDA's ability to safeguard the public by allowing harm to occur before action can be taken to protect the public. As to the safety of these products "caveat emptor" is the rule of the day—the exact opposite of what the consumers assume is the case. Surveys of older Americans find that approximately 75 percent want the government to review and approve supplements for safety and verify all marketing claims *before* they are sold in the market.[7] In many ways we have returned to pre-1906 legislation days when unproven and harmful patent medicines and cures were rampant.

While dietary supplement makers have enjoyed deregulation of supplements in recent years, they are beginning to experience repercussions. Media reports deriding supplement safety are increasing. Press coverage regarding the difficulties the FDA encountered when trying to ban ephedra supplements, even after numerous reports of adverse events and death, has been increasing. The National Nutritional Foods Association (NNFA), recognizing this increasing negative focus on supplement safety, supported the Dietary Supplement and Nonprescription Drug Consumer Protection Act,[8] which puts some responsibility for safety back onto the manufacturer by requiring them to notify FDA about life-threatening events, hospitalizations, significant disabilities, birth defects, and medical interventions caused by their products. A contact number is now required on all labels should customers need to report problems.

Consumers themselves are also beginning to realize that many claims made about supplements and functional foods are marketing "hype" designed to increase product sales and manufacturer bottom lines, not necessarily to improve the health and safety of the consumer. Judy Foreman, a writer for the *Boston Globe*, sums up this growing disenchantment with supplements in her May 14, 2007 "Health Sense" column. She writes her "love affair with vitamins and supplements is over: with a few exceptions . . . I'm tossing them out." She further explains that reports about vitamins and minerals influenced her to take specific supplements, mostly antioxidants. But as scientific studies began to accumulate disputing previous claims of improved health or showed they could be dangerous, she stopped taking most of them. She does admit that multivitamins will remain a part of her daily regime for now because she fails to eat enough fruits and vegetables. But even this has her concerned after reading the recent ConsumerLab.com analysis that revealed many multivitamins are either contaminated with lead, do not dissolve properly, or do not contain the ingredients or amounts listed on the label. She notes one benefit of not taking these supplements is "the handful of twenties I'm not spending on supplements!"[9]

An article in the *Chicago Tribune* on April 19, 2007[10] reports Kraft Foods Inc. has identified functional foods, which are highly profitable, as the next product line they will be focusing on to improve their decreasing profit margins. Coca-Cola and PepsiCo, responding to decreasing soft drink sales, plan on introducing carbonated beverages fortified with vitamins and minerals (and

Table 6.2
Nutrient Composition of Select Functional Foods

Nutrient/serving	CocaVia, Original Chocolate Bar	Kellogg's *SmartStart Antioxidant* Cereal (no milk)	Kellogg's Cornflakes (no milk)
Calories	100	190	100
Vitamin A	<2%	25% (10% as beta carotene)	10%
Vitamin C	15%	25%	10%
Calcium	25%	0%	0%
Iron	4%	100%	45%
Vitamin D	–	10%	10%
Vitamin E	20%	100%	–
Thiamin	–	100%	25%
Riboflavin	–	100%	25%
Niacin	–	100%	25%
Vitamin B_6	15%	100%	25%
Folic Acid	15%	100%	25%
Vitamin B_{12}	15%	100%	25%
Panthothenate	–	100%	–
Phosphorus	–	8%	–
Magnesium	–	6%	–
Zinc	–	100%	–

Note: Values listed are the percent of the daily value (DV) for a healthy adult in one serving of this food. In general, 5 percent or less is considered low and 20 percent and above is considered high. For example, Kellogg's Cornflakes provides only 10 percent of the recommended daily value (% DV) for vitamin A based on a 2000 calorie daily diet. So if you ate approximately 2000 calories per day to keep your weight stable, you would only get 10 percent of your daily RDA for vitamin A from one serving of cornflakes and thus need to include other vitamin A food sources in that day's diet. If caloric needs are less, then even less of the DV would be taken in.
Source: Adapted from Kellogg's corporate Web site at http://www2.kelloggs.com/Product/Product.aspx; dietfacts.com at http://www.dietfacts.com.

no calories) in the spring of 2007.[11] Kellogg's *Smart Start Antioxidants* cereal promises to "give your immune system a little help to work hard for you. With Vitamin A (including beta carotene), Vitamin C, Vitamin E, and zinc, *Smart Start Antioxidants* cereal is a serious combination of antioxidant protection."[12] Mars, Inc. introduced it's CocoaVia Heart Healthy Snacks via the Internet in 2005 and retail stores in 2006. As CocoaVia's marketing information tells us, they are "tasty chocolate treats" that have a "twist of health" because of a production process that is "designed to protect and maintain the high levels of the naturally occurring cocoa flavanols."[13] As Table 6.2 highlights, one serving of *Smart Start Antioxidants* cereal contains 100 percent of most important nutrients in the daily diet.

CocoaVia contains few nutrients in a 100 calorie portion size, claims benefits yet to be proven from flavanols, and also contains cholesterol-lowering sterols and stanols, which may interfere with absorption of ß-carotene and vitamin E. So even though ß-carotene and vitamin E are added nutrients, their absorption may possibly be negated by the stanols and sterols in this expensive functional food/nutraceutical. As these illustrations highlight, unless the daily diet is carefully planned, the potential for nutrient interactions and excess intakes is substantial. These products are just the tip of the iceberg. As food manufacturers enhance foods to enter the functional foods/nutraceuticals market, concerns about "hypersupplementation" will rise. The majority of supplement users are better educated, have higher incomes, are older, and take an active and preventive approach toward their health. However, as we have seen, antioxidant vitamin and mineral intakes from the available American diet provide sufficient, and at times more than, DRI levels of these essential micronutrients. In addition, dietary supplements and functional foods/nutraceuticals support the concept that food is medicine and may sway individuals from eating a balanced diet from natural food sources believing that they can acquire the same or superior benefits from supplementation at a lower overall cost. Instead of improving eating patterns to include more fruits, vegetables, and whole grains, people tend to eat the same foods they have always eaten (often processed and high in sugars and fats) with the "insurance" of a supplement to "fix" all that is wrong with their diet. Aging Americans, who also tend to have an increased use of pharmaceutical medications, have a tendency to incorporate supplements and functional foods/nutraceuticals into what may already be a nutritionally adequate diet. Nutrient and drug interactions, toxicities, and overdoses may contribute to a potential public safety disaster.

ANTIOXIDANT GUIDELINES

The antioxidant nutrients—vitamins C and E, carotenoids, selenium, and polyphenols—do appear to have a positive correlation in chronic disease reduction and better overall health. But lifestyle factors (exercise, tobacco and alcohol use, and diet choices key among them) and genetic factors also factor heavily into disease incidence. Scientific evidence is insufficient to prove that antioxidant nutrients are the exclusive reason for benefits observed from high phytochemical intake of fruits and vegetables. Antioxidants also do not appear to be a quick fix in prevention or treatment of chronic health problems that may have taken decades to develop, despite the hopes of so many Americans. As we discussed earlier in this book, the NIH concluded in their 2006 State of the Science Multivitamin/Mineral Supplements and Chronic Disease conference[14] that:

1. More accurate information is needed about dietary supplement use in the population and study methods need to be improved.
2. Dietary supplement databases need to be built with ingredient information and regular updates.

3. Effective communication methods to disseminate scientific information to the public is needed.
4. Dietary supplement and medication interactions must be studied.
5. Population segments, previously underrepresented and at risk for chronic disease, need to be studied.
6. New biomedical sciences, such as nutrigenomics, need to be studied and techniques applied to observational and randomized, controlled, clinical studies.
7. Efficacy and safety of individual vitamins, minerals and vitamin/mineral combinations need to be studied more rigorously.

While all of these are worthy recommendations and should be implemented, gathering information via studies and setting up informational databases takes time and utilizes scarce resources. In the meantime, the average consumer and health care professional continues to be uncertain about just what to do when it comes to antioxidants. So just what should we do about them?

The leading causes of death in the United States—coronary heart disease, cancer, stroke, and diabetes—have been associated with poor diet choices.[15] Many positive health outcomes have been associated with increasing dietary intake of fruits, vegetables, legumes, and whole grains—all high in naturally occurring antioxidant nutrients. Combining different fruits and vegetables has also been discovered to have an even greater disease-fighting potential (for example, mixing tomatoes with broccoli instead of consuming separately has been shown to provide a much more potent combination in prostate cancer reduction).[16] In 1991, the National Cancer Institute and the Produce for Better Health Foundation partnered to create the 5 A Day For Better Health Program. The 5 A Day Program focuses on increasing public awareness about eating a diet high in fruits and vegetables for better health and reduction of stroke, high blood pressure, diabetes, and cancer risks. Despite this national marketing effort, fruit and vegetable consumption appears to have remained below recommended levels. The *Healthy People 2010* objectives for our nation recommended increasing fruit and vegetable consumption of at least two daily servings of fruit to 75 percent of the population, and at least three daily servings of vegetables to 50 percent of the population. But *The State of Aging and Health in America 2007* Report, which is submitted by the CDC, learned that approximately 29.8 percent of all Americans are currently meeting these goals. However, a *Journal of the American Dietetic Association* study, using data from the NHANES 1999–2000 and 1994–1996 CSFII, reported 40 percent of Americans ate the recommended amount of at least five servings of fruits and vegetables daily between 1999 to 2000.[17] Despite these discrepancies in study results, which highlight just how difficult it is to really accurately assess food and nutrient intakes, the bottom line still reveals that Americans continue to eat below optimal levels of fruits and vegetables (although consumption was estimated to have increased by 3 percent between 1990 and 2000).[18] Cultural food preferences, environmental barriers, cost, convenience, advertising, and lack of education are just some of the barriers affecting fruit and vegetable consumption in the United States.

The clearest answer about what to do when advising others about antioxidants appears to be what mothers and home economic teachers have recommended for years: eat a healthy and well-balanced diet with an emphasis on intake of fruits, vegetables, legumes, and whole grains. Obviously, exercise and lifestyle habits (avoiding tobacco, alcohol, and drug abuse) and genetic legacy factor into our prospective overall health. But controlling what we eat and making healthy, nutrient-dense food choices (*not* gulping down a dietary supplement pill in place of them) appears to be the best choice when trying to prevent or delay chronic illnesses and improve quality of life as we age.

It should be kept in mind, however, that there is a function and role for dietary supplements. Specific at-risk populations—such as those who live in poverty, the elderly who have changing gastric secretions that may affect how much of a nutrient is absorbed, those consuming below 1,600 calories per day, and those who suffer from diseases that affect nutrient absorption—benefit from supervised dietary supplementation. Supplements are a relatively inexpensive form of nutrients that can be administered, if taken consistently, in a more precise and reliable dose than through fruits and vegetables. As such, they may be beneficial for certain life stage groups, such as during pregnancy and the elderly years when appetite and nutrient intake or absorption are diminished.

Based on the growing body of evidence that using foods to meet nutrient needs is safer and more beneficial to our health, the Department of Health and Human Services (HHS) and the USDA published dietary guidelines that promote health and reduce risk for chronic disease. These guidelines, reviewed every five years, take into account current research and the state of health in America, seeking to provide an overall pattern of eating that will improve health and that the general public can easily follow. The *Dietary Guidelines for Americans 2005*[19] promotes the need for all healthy Americans to choose meals and snacks high in variety and that are nutrient-dense but low in excess calories, saturated and trans fat, added sugars, and alcohol. At-risk populations have specific nutrition risks. People over age 50 are often low in vitamin B_{12}, pregnant women are often low in iron, women of childbearing age need to fortify their daily diet with folic acid (from functional foods or supplements) to prevent birth defects, and older adults or people who are dark skinned (or get very little exposure to sunlight) are often deficient in vitamin D. HHS and USDA recommends two food guides for better health: the USDA Food Guide and the DASH Eating Plan. These guides allow individuals to meet their daily DRIs without the need of additional supplementation. But if a person's diet is not varied, doesn't include enough fruits, vegetables, and whole grains, or is below 1,600 calories, then functional foods or multivitamins may be of benefit.

In general, it appears that most American adults consume less than recommended amounts of calcium, potassium, fiber, magnesium, and vitamins A (carotenoids), C, and E even though the IOM draws different conclusions.

Table 6.3
Sample USDA Food Guide and the DASH Eating Plan at the 2,000-Calorie Level[a]

Food Groups and Subgroups	USDA Food Guide Amount[b]	DASH Eating Plan Amount	Equivalent Amounts
Fruit Group	2 cups (4 servings)	2 to 2.5 cups (4 to 5 servings)	1/2 cup equivalent is: 1/2 cup fresh, frozen, or canned fruit; 1 med fruit; 1/4 cup dried fruit; 1/2 cup fruit juice
Vegetable Group		2 to 2.5 cups (4 to 5 servings)	1/2 cup equivalent is: 1/2 cup of cut-up raw or cooked vegetable; 1 cup raw leafy vegetable; 1/2 cup vegetable juice
Dark green vegetables	2.5 cups (5 servings)		
Orange vegetables	3 cups/week		
Legumes (dry beans)	2 cups/week		
Starchy vegetables	3 cups/week		
Other vegetables	3 cups/week		
	6.5 cups/week		
Grain Group	6 ounce-equivalents	6 to 8 ounce-equivalents (6 to 8 servings)	1 ounce-equivalent is: 1 slice bread; 1 cup dry cereal; 1/2 cup cooked rice, pasta, cereal; DASH: 1 oz dry cereal (1/2–1 1/4 cup depending on cereal type—check label)
Whole grains	3 ounce-equivalents		
Other grains	3 ounce-equivalents		
Meat and Beans Group	5.5 ounce-equivalents	6 ounces or less meats, poultry, fish; 4 to 5 servings per week nuts, seeds, and legumes[d]	1 ounce-equivalent is: 1 ounce of cooked lean meats, poultry, fish; 1 egg[e]; USDA: 1/4 cup cooked dry beans or tofu, 1 Tbsp peanut butter, 1/2 oz nuts or seeds; DASH: 1 1/2 oz nuts, 2 Tbsp peanut butter, 1/2 oz seeds, 1/2 cup cooked dry beans

Milk Group	3 cups	2 to 3 cups	1 cup equivalent is: 1 cup low-fat/fat-free milk, yogurt 1½ oz of low-fat, fat-free, or reduced fat natural cheese 2 oz of low-fat or fat-free processed cheese
Oils	27 grams (6 tsp)	8 to 12 grams (2 to 3 tsp)	DASH: 1 tsp equivalent is: 1 tsp soft margarine 1 Tbsp low-fat mayo 2 Tbsp light salad dressing 1 tsp vegetable oil
Discretionary Calorie Allowance	267 calories		
Example of distribution:			
Solid fat[f]	18 grams		
Added sugars	8 tsp	~2 tsp of added sugar (5 Tbsp per week)	DASH: 1 Tbsp added sugar equivalent is: 1 Tbsp jelly or jam ½ cup sorbet and ices 1 cup lemonade

Note: Table updated to reflect 2006 DASH Eating Plan. Amounts of various food groups that are recommended each day or each week in the USDA Food Guide and in the DASH Eating Plan (amounts are daily unless otherwise specified) at the 2,000-calorie level. Also identified are equivalent amounts for different food choices in each group. To follow either eating pattern, food choices over time should provide these amounts of food from each group on average.

[a] All servings are per day unless otherwise noted. USDA vegetable subgroup amounts and amounts of DASH nuts, seeds, and dry beans are per week.

[b] The 2,000-calorie USDA Food Guide is appropriate for many sedentary males 51 to 70 years of age, sedentary females 19 to 30 years of age, and for some other gender/age groups who are more physically active. See table 3 for information about gender/age/activity levels and appropriate calorie intakes. Whole grains are recommended for most grain servings to meet fiber recommendations.

[c] Whole grains are recommended for most grain servings to meet fiber recommendations.

[d] In the DASH Eating Plan, nuts, seeds, and legumes are a separate food group from meats, poultry, and fish.

[e] Since eggs are high in cholesterol, limit egg yolk intake to no more than 4 per week; 2 egg whites have the same protein content as 1 oz of meat.

[f] The oils listed in this table are not considered to be part of discretionary calories because they are a major source of the vitamin E and polyunsaturated fatty acids, including the essential fatty acids, in the food pattern. In contrast, solid fats (i.e., saturated and *trans* fats) are listed separately as a source of discretionary calories.

Source: USDA and HHS, "Dietary Guidelines for Americans 2005," Chapter 2, Table 1; http://www.health.gov/dietaryguidelines/dga2005/document/html/chapter2.htm#table2.

Children and adolescents consume less than recommended amounts of calcium, potassium, fiber, magnesium, and vitamin E. At-risk populations (as mentioned previously) tend to consume less of vitamin B_{12}, iron, folic acid, and vitamins E and D. Americans generally consume too many calories and too much saturated fat, cholesterol, added sugars, and salt. The first key point the USDA Food Guide and the DASH Eating Plans stress is the inclusion of more dark green and orange vegetables, fruits, legumes, whole grains, and low-fat milk and milk products and less refined grains, total fats, added sugars, and calories in the daily diet. The second point they stress is picking foods that are nutrient-dense. Nutrient-dense foods provide substantial amounts of vitamins and minerals in few calories. For example, fruits and vegetables are nutrient-dense foods because they contain antioxidants (vitamins, minerals, and phytochemicals) and fiber at low calorie levels. In comparison, processed foods often high in sugar, fat, and salt—such as cookies and potato chips—are poor nutrient-dense food choices because they contain very little (and sometimes no) nutrient values at a high calorie level. The two diet plans are very similar but the DASH plan is lower in sodium than the USDA Food Guide. Table 6.3 and Table 6.4 outline the USDA Food Guide and DASH Eating Plan eating patterns for a 2,000-calorie diet and compare them against the DRIs.[20]

In addition to the HHS and USDA dietary guidelines, the CDC partners with other government agencies and not-for-profit and industry groups to increase public awareness about the benefits of fruits and vegetables and increasing their consumption through the National Fruit & Vegetable Program (formerly the 5 A Day For Better Health Program). They support the HHS and USDA dietary guidelines and provide a Web site, listed in Appendix C, which helps people learn about the benefits of eating these natural antioxidants and also gives tips, ideas, and recipes to assist people to increase them in their diet.[21] Individuals may also want to incorporate more organic produce into their diets as well. Although more expensive, one study indicates their value may be worth the extra expense. Studies are still ongoing to determine whether there is a significant difference between organic and conventional produce. Nevertheless, organic products are becoming more popular and available. As demand continues to increase, more suppliers will enter the market and prices should come down.

In general, all vitamin and mineral needs should be consumed via natural food sources. But because most Americans do not eat the recommended amounts of fruits and vegetables, eat on the run (therefore eating at fast food restaurants or not balancing meals), and/or follow weight-reducing diets, taking a multivitamin/multimineral is an appropriate choice to compensate for possible nutrient deficits in the diet. To date the evidence neither supports nor opposes taking a daily multivitamin as "insurance."[22] Even if a healthy diet is eaten, which follows all recommendations, taking an additional multivitamin/multimineral supplement as an inexpensive "insurance" is unlikely to

Table 6.4
Comparison of Selected Nutrients in the Dietary Approaches to Stop
Hypertension (DASH) Eating Plan[a], the USDA Food Guide[b], and Nutrient
Intakes Recommended Per Day by the Institute of Medicine (IOM)[c]

Nutrient	DASH Eating Plan (2,000 kcals)	USDA Food Guide (2,000 kcals)	IOM Recommendations for Females 19 to 30
Protein, g	105	91	RDA: 46
Protein, % kcal	20	18	AMDR: 10–35
Carbohydrate, g	281	271	RDA: 130
Carbohydrate, % kcal	54	55	AMDR: 45–65
Total fat, g	60	65	–
Total fat, % kcal	26	29	AMDR: 20–35
Saturated fat, g	12	17	–
Saturated fat, % kcal	6	7.8	ALAP[d]
Monounsaturated fat, g	25	24	–
Monounsaturated fat, % kcal	12	11	–
Polyunsaturated fat, g	16	20	–
Polyunsaturated fat, % kcal	7	9.0	–
Linoleic acid, g	14	18	AI: 12
Alpha-linolenic acid, g	2.2	1.7	AI: 1.1
Cholesterol, mg	136	230	ALAP[d]
Total dietary fiber, g	34	31	AI: 28[e]
Potassium, mg	4,721	4,044	AI: 4,700
Sodium, mg	2,096[f]	1,779	AI: 1,500, UL: <2,300
Calcium, mg	1,406	1,316	AI: 1,000
Magnesium, mg	554	380	RDA: 310
Copper, mg	1.9	1.5	RDA: 0.9
Iron, mg	22	18	RDA: 18
Phosphorus, mg	1,955	1,740	RDA: 700
Zinc, mg	14	14	RDA: 8
Thiamin, mg	1.7	2.0	RDA: 1.1
Riboflavin, mg	2.7	2.8	RDA: 1.1
Niacin equivalents, mg	50	22	RDA: 14
Vitamin B_6, mg	2.9	2.4	RDA: 1.3
Vitamin B_{12}, μg	5.6	8.3	RDA: 2.4
Vitamin C, mg	162	155	RDA: 75
Vitamin E (AT)[g]	19	9.5	RDA: 15.0
Vitamin A, μg (RAE)[h]	925	1,052	RDA: 700

Table 6.4 *(continued)*

Note: Table updated to reflect 2006 DASH Eating Plan. Estimated nutrient levels in the DASH Eating Plan and the USDA Food Guide at the 2,000-calorie level, as well as the nutrient intake levels recommended by the Institute of Medicine (IOM) for females 19–30 years of age.

[a] DASH nutrient values are based on a 1-week menu of the DASH Eating Plan. Visit www. nhlbi.nih.gov.

[b] USDA nutrient values are based on population-weighted averages of typical food choices within each food group or subgroup.

[c] Recommended intakes for adult females 19–30; RDA = Recommended Dietary Allowance; AI = Adequate Intake; AMDR = Acceptable Macronutrient Distribution Range; UL = Upper Limit.

[d] As low as possible while consuming a nutritionally adequate diet.

[e] Amount listed is based on 14 g dietary fiber/1,000 kcal.

[f] The DASH Eating Plan also can be used to follow at 1,500 mg sodium per day.

[g] AT = mg d-α-tocopherol.

[h] RAE = Retinol Activity Equivalents.

Source: USDA and HHS, "Dietary Guidelines for Americans 2005," Chapter 2, Table 2; http://www.health.gov/dietaryguidelines/dga2005/document/html/chapter2.htm#table2.

exceed the ULs for nutrients. Table 6.5 lists nutrients and amounts (both minimums and maximums) that represent an adequate multivitamin supplement. Additionally, natural or synthetic brands make no difference in absorption of most nutrients and it is best to purchase the least expensive brand that is free of fillers and other additives (such as sugar, yeast, or artificial colorings) that conform to U.S. Pharmacopeia (USP) guidelines. Multivitamin/multimineral supplements should be taken within thirty minutes before or after meals.

Concerns about quality of multivitamins on the market surfaced when a recent ConsumerLab.com analysis found some products were contaminated with lead, did not have the correct amounts of listed nutrients, and/or did not dissolve properly.[23] (Both ConsumerLab.com and the USP are independent agencies that test health products and pharmaceuticals, including supplements.) This study supports the concept that ingesting daily nutrients from foods is the best option.

However, adding functional foods/nutraceuticals and multivitamins/multiminerals to adequate diets may become problematic and may lead to hypersupplementation. As we saw with one nutraceutical that provided 100 percent of most daily nutrients (Kellogg's *SmartStart Antioxidant* Cereal), including this cereal every day along with a balanced and adequate diet plus a multivitamin/multimineral can quite possibly lead to taking in excess recommended nutrient intakes.

When considering functional foods/nutraceuticals, the following questions should be asked before consuming them:

> *Should I be eating this?* Don't add this food just for its medicinal value.
>
> *How meaningful is the claim?* When a product claims that it affects the body, that is, "supports the immune system" or "enhances mood," what scientific evidence backs up the claim? Beware ORAC (oxygen radical absorbance capacity) claims. Marketers often suggest a high ORAC value "proves" superior

Table 6.5
What to Look for in a Multivitamin/Multimineral Supplement

Nutrient	RDA* for adults	UL*
Vitamin A	700–900 µgRAE*/d	2,800–3,000 µgRAE*/d
Vitamin C	75–90 mg/d	2,000 mg/d
Vitamin D (cholecalciferol)	AI*: 5–15 µg/d	50 µg/d
Vitamin E (d-alpha tocopherol)	15 mg/d	1,000 mg/d
Vitamin B_1 (thiamine)	1.1–1.2 mg/d	none
Vitamin B_2 (riboflavin)	1.1–1.3 mg/d	none
Vitamin B_3 (niacin)	14–16 mg/d	35 mg/d
Vitamin B_6 (pyridoxine)	1.3–1.7 mg/d	100 mg/d
Folate (folic acid)	400 µg/d	1000 µg/d
Vitamin B_{12} (cobalamin)	2.4 µg/d	none
Vitamin K	AI*: 90–120 µg/d	none
Biotin	AI*: 30 µg/d	none
Calcium (citrate or carbonate)	AI*: 1,000–1,200 mg/d	2,500 mg/d
Chromium	AI*: 20–35 µg/d	none
Copper	900 µg/d	10,000 µg/d
Iron	8–18 mg/d	45 mg/d
Magnesium	310–420 mg/d	350 mg/d
Manganese	AI*: 1.8–2.3 mg/d	11 mg/d
Molybdenum	43–45 µg/d	2,000 µg/d
Pantothenic Acid	AI*: 5 mg/d	none
Phosphorus	700 mg/d	4,000 mg/d
Selenium	55 µg/d	400 µg/d
Zinc	8–11 mg/d	40 mg/d

Note: *RAE = retinol activity equivalent; RDA = Recommended Dietary Allowance for adults 19 years and older; AI = Adequate Intake; UL = Tolerable Upper Intake Level.
Source: Adapted from Otten, *Dietary Reference Intakes, The Essential Guide to Nutrient Requirements* (2006).

antioxidant value. The ORAC assay, however, is only one of many assays that measure the capability of a product or food to "quench radicals" and are useful in the lab setting and in vitro *only.* All these assays, including the ORAC, are limited and none truly measure "radical quenching" of all radicals. They do not predict health effects of antioxidants in humans. Marketing claims about product antioxidant capacity are often overstated, unscientific, and written out of context.

Do I need this(these) nutrient(s)? Healthy people who eat well-balanced diets do not need to add these products to their diet. If an individual is in an at-risk category or has diseases that may affect nutrient absorption, then their diet must be carefully evaluated before adding them into a daily diet.

Am I overdosing? Be sure to know what the maximum amount of any nutrient is safe to take and the sources of the nutrient to avoid toxicities.

As we explored throughout this book, there is some evidence that free radicals can cause oxidative damage to cells. Antioxidants appear to reduce this damage and are worth incorporating into our daily diets, although supporting evidence has been conflicting. But the source of antioxidants should come from a balanced diet that includes a variety of fruits, vegetables, legumes, and whole grains. Much more research needs to be done and the media and the average American need to take a wait-and-see approach, rather than jump on the latest fad, which could endanger their health. The media should also give more publicity to the government programs that have been already been put into place to help Americans improve their health. Lastly, health care professionals need to be better informed about current self-care trends that Americans are embracing and actively query their patients about what they are doing, educating them on the benefits and dangers. Hippocrates seems to have summed it up best:

Let food be thy medicine, thy medicine shall be thy food.

—Hippocrates[24]

APPENDICES

Appendix A
Dietary Reference Intakes (DRI)–2000 for Life Stage Groups

Water-soluble Vitamins

Thiamin (Vt. B₁) (mg/d)

	0–6 mths	7–12 mths	1–3 yrs	4–8 yrs	9–13 yrs	14–18 yrs	19–30 yrs	31–50 yrs	51–70 yrs	>70 yrs	Pregnancy <18 yrs	19–50 yrs	Lactation <18 yrs	19–50 yrs
EAR	–	–	0.4	0.5	0.7	Male 1.0 / Female 0.9	Male 1.0 / Female 0.9	Male 1.0 / Female 0.9	Male 1.0 / Female 0.9	Male 1.0 / Female 0.9	1.2	1.2	1.2	1.2
RDA	–	–	0.5	0.6	0.9	Male 1.2 / Female 1.0	Male 1.2 / Female 1.1	Male 1.2 / Female 1.1	Male 1.2 / Female 1.1	Male 1.2 / Female 1.1	1.4	1.4	1.4	1.4
AI	0.2	0.3	–	–	–	–	–	–	–	–	–	–	–	–
UL	–	–	–	–	–	–	–	–	–	–	–	–	–	–

Riboflavin (Vt. B₂) (mg/d)

	0–6 mths	7–12 mths	1–3 yrs	4–8 yrs	9–13 yrs	14–18 yrs	19–30 yrs	31–50 yrs	51–70 yrs	>70 yrs	Pregnancy <18 yrs	19–50 yrs	Lactation <18 yrs	19–50 yrs
EAR	–	–	0.4	0.5	0.8	Male 1.1 / Female 0.9	Male 1.1 / Female 0.9	Male 1.1 / Female 0.9	Male 1.1 / Female 0.9	Male 1.1 / Female 0.9	1.2	1.2	1.3	1.3
RDA	–	–	0.5	0.6	0.9	Male 1.3 / Female 1.0	Male 1.3 / Female 1.1	Male 1.3 / Female 1.1	Male 1.3 / Female 1.1	Male 1.3 / Female 1.1	1.4	1.4	1.6	1.6
AI	0.3	0.4	–	–	–	–	–	–	–	–	–	–	–	–
UL	–	–	–	–	–	–	–	–	–	–	–	–	–	–

Niacin (Vt. B₃) (mg/d)

EAR	–	–	5	6	9	Male 12 / Female 11	Male 12 / Female 11	Male 12 / Female 11	Male 12 / Female 11	14	14	13	13
RDA	–	–	6	8	12	Male 16 / Female 14	Male 16 / Female 14	Male 16 / Female 14	Male 16 / Female 14	18	18	17	17
AI	2	4	–	–	–	–	–	–	–	–	–	–	–
UL	ND	ND	10	15	20	30	35	35	35	30	35	30	35

Vitamin B₆ (mg/d)

EAR	–	–	0.4	0.5	0.8	Male 1.1 / Female 1.0	Male 1.1 / Female 1.1	Male 1.4 / Female 1.3	Male 1.4 / Female 1.3	1.6	1.6	1.7	1.7
RDA	–	–	0.5	0.6	1.0	Male 1.3 / Female 1.2	Male 1.3 / Female 1.3	Male 1.7 / Female 1.5	Male 1.7 / Female 1.5	1.9	1.9	2.0	2.0
AI	0.1	0.3	–	–	–	–	–	–	–	–	–	–	–
UL	ND	ND	30	40	60	80	100	100	100	80	100	80	100

Folate (μg/d)

EAR	–	–	120	160	250	330	320	320	320	520	520	450	450
RDA	–	–	150	200	300	400	400	400	400	600	600	500	500
AI	65	80	–	–	–	–	–	–	–	–	–	–	–
UL	ND	ND	300	400	600	800	1,000	1,000	1,000	800	1,000	800	1,000

(Continued)

119

Appendix A (Continued)

	0–6 mths	7–12 mths	1–3 yrs	4–8 yrs	9–13 yrs	14–18 yrs	19–30 yrs	31–50 yrs	51–70 yrs	>70 yrs	Pregnancy <18 yrs	19–50 yrs	Lactation <18 yrs	19–50 yrs
Vitamin B$_{12}$ (µg/d)														
EAR	–	–	0.7	1.0	1.5	2.0	2.0	2.0	2.0	2.0	2.2	2.2	2.4	2.4
RDA	–	–	0.9	1.2	1.8	2.4	2.4	2.4	2.4	2.4	2.6	2.6	2.8	2.8
AI	0.4	0.5	–	–	–	–	–	–	–	–	–	–	–	–
UL	–	–	–	–	–	–	–	–	–	–	–	–	–	–
Fat-soluble Vitamins														
Vitamin D (µg/d)														
AI	5	5	5	5	5	5	5	5	10	15	5	5	5	5
UL	25	25	50	50	50	50	50	50	50	50	50	50	50	50
Vitamin K (µg/d)														
AI	2.0	2.5	30	55	60	75	Male 120 Female 90	Male 120 Female 90	Male 120 Female 90	Male 120 Female 90	75	90	75	90
Vitamin Co-enzymes														
Biotin (µg/d)														
AI	5	6	8	12	20	25	30	30	30	30	30	30	35	35
Choline (mg/d)														
AI	125	150	200	250	375	Male 550 Female 400	Male 550 Female 425	Male 550 Female 425	Male 550 Female 425	Male 550 Female 425	450	450	550	550
UL	ND	ND	1,000	1,000	2,000	3,000	3,500	3,500	3,500	3,500	3,000	3,500	3,000	3,500

Pantothenic Acid (mg/d)

Measure														
AI	1.7	1.8	2	3	4	5	5	5	5	5	6	6	7	7

Minerals

Calcium (mg/d)

Measure														
AI	210	270	500	800	1,300	1,300	1,000	1,000	1,200	1,200	1,300	1,000	1,300	1,000
UL	ND	ND	2,500	2,500	2,500	2,500	2,500	2,500	2,500	2,500	2,500	2,500	2,500	2,500

Chromium (μg/d)

Measure														
AI	0.2	5.5	11	15	**Male** 25 / **Female** 21	**Male** 35 / **Female** 24	**Male** 35 / **Female** 25	**Male** 35 / **Female** 25	**Male** 30 / **Female** 20	**Male** 30 / **Female** 20	29	30	44	45

Copper (μg/d)

Measure														
EAR	–	–	260	340	540	685	700	700	700	700	785	800	985	1,000
RDA	–	–	340	440	700	890	900	900	900	900	1,000	1,000	1,300	1,300
AI	200	220	–	–	–	–	–	–	–	–	–	–	–	–
UL	ND	ND	1,000	3,000	5,000	8,000	10,000	10,000	10,000	10,000	8,000	10,000	8,000	10,000

Potassium (g/d)

Measure														
AI	0.4	0.7	3.0	3.8	4.5	4.7	4.7	4.7	4.7	4.7	4.7	4.7	5.1	5.1

Vanadium (mg/d)

Measure														
UL	ND	ND	ND	ND	ND	ND	1.8	1.8	1.8	1.8	ND	ND	ND	ND

121

(Continued)

Appendix A (Continued)

Fluoride (mg/d)

	0–6 mths	7–12 mths	1–3 yrs	4–8 yrs	9–13 yrs	14–18 yrs	19–30 yrs	31–50 yrs	51–70 yrs	>70 yrs	Pregnancy <18 yrs	19–50 yrs	Lactation <18 yrs	19–50 yrs
AI	0.01	0.5	0.7	1.0	2.0	3	Male 4 / Female 3	Male 4 / Female 3	Male 4 / Female 3	Male 4 / Female 3	3	3	3	3
UL	0.7	0.9	1.3	2.2	10	10	10	10	10	10	10	10	10	10

Iodine (µg/d)

	0–6 mths	7–12 mths	1–3 yrs	4–8 yrs	9–13 yrs	14–18 yrs	19–30 yrs	31–50 yrs	51–70 yrs	>70 yrs	Pregnancy <18 yrs	19–50 yrs	Lactation <18 yrs	19–50 yrs
EAR	–	–	65	65	73	95	95	95	95	95	160	160	209	209
RDA	–	–	90	90	120	150	150	150	150	150	220	220	290	290
AI	110	130	–	–	–	–	–	–	–	–	–	–	–	–
UL	ND	ND	200	300	600	900	1,100	1,100	1,100	1,100	900	1,100	900	1,100

Iron (mg/d)

	0–6 mths	7–12 mths	1–3 yrs	4–8 yrs	9–13 yrs	14–18 yrs	19–30 yrs	31–50 yrs	51–70 yrs	>70 yrs	Pregnancy <18 yrs	19–50 yrs	Lactation <18 yrs	19–50 yrs
EAR	–	6.9	3.0	4.1	Male 5.9 / Female 5.7	Male 7.7 / Female 7.9	Male 6.0 / Female 8.1	Male 6.0 / Female 8.1	Male 6.0 / Female 5.0	Male 6.0 / Female 5.0	23	22	7	6.5
RDA	–	11	7	10	8	Male 11 / Female 15	Male 8 / Female 18	Male 8 / Female 18	Male 8 / Female 8	Male 8 / Female 8	27	27	10	9
AI	0.27	–	–	–	–	–	–	–	–	–	–	–	–	–
UL	40	40	40	40	40	45	45	45	45	45	45	45	45	45

Boron (mg/d)

	1	2	3	4	5	6	7	8	9	10	11	12	13	14
UL	ND	ND	3	6	11	17	20	20	20	20	17	20	17	20

Magnesium (mg/d)

	1	2	3	4	5	6	7	8	9	10	11	12	13	14
EAR	–	–	65	110	200	Male 340 / Female 300	Male 330 / Female 255	Male 350 / Female 265	Male 350 / Female 265	Male 350 / Female 265	335	290–300	300	255–265
RDA	–	–	80	130	240	Male 410 / Female 360	Male 400 / Female 310	Male 420 / Female 320	Male 420 / Female 320	Male 420 / Female 320	400	350–360	360	310–320
AI	30	75	–	–	–	–	–	–	–	–	–	–	–	–
UL	ND	ND	65	110	350	350	350	350	350	350	350	350	350	350

Manganese (mg/d)

	1	2	3	4	5	6	7	8	9	10	11	12	13	14
AI	0.003	0.6	1.2	1.5	Male 1.9 / Female 1.6	Male 2.2 / Female 1.6	Male 2.3 / Female 1.8	Male 2.3 / Female 1.8	Male 2.3 / Female 1.8	Male 2.3 / Female 1.8	2	2	2.6	2.6
UL	ND	ND	2	3	6	9	11	11	11	11	9	11	9	11

Molybdenum (µg/d)

	1	2	3	4	5	6	7	8	9	10	11	12	13	14
EAR	–	–	13	17	26	33	34	34	34	34	40	40	35	36
RDA	–	–	17	22	34	43	45	45	45	45	50	50	50	50
AI	2	3	–	–	–	–	–	–	–	–	–	–	–	–
UL	ND	ND	300	600	1,100	1,700	2,000	2,000	2,000	2,000	1,700	2,000	1,700	2,000

Nickel (mg/d)

	1	2	3	4	5	6	7	8	9	10	11	12	13	14
UL	ND	ND	0.2	0.3	0.6	1.0	1.0	1.0	1.0	1.0	1.0	1.0	1.0	1.0

(Continued)

Appendix A *(Continued)*

	0–6 mths	7–12 mths	1–3 yrs	4–8 yrs	9–13 yrs	14–18 yrs	19–30 yrs	31–50 yrs	51–70 yrs	>70 yrs	Pregnancy <18 yrs	19–50 yrs	Lactation <18 yrs	19–50 yrs
Phosphorus (mg/d)														
EAR	–	–	380	405	1,055	1,055	580	580	580	580	1,005	580	1,005	580
RDA	–	–	460	500	1,250	1,250	700	700	700	700	1,250	700	1,250	700
AI	100	275	–	–	–	–	–	–	–	–	–	–	–	–
UL	ND	ND	3,000	3,000	4,000	4,000	4,000	4,000	4,000	3,000	3,500	3,500	4,000	4,000
Sodium (g/d)														
AI	0.12	0.37	1.0	1.2	1.5	1.5	1.5	1.5	1.3	1.2	1.5	1.5	1.5	1.5
UL	ND	ND	1.5	1.9	2.2	2.3	2.3	2.3	2.3	2.3	2.3	2.3	2.3	2.3
Chloride (g/d)														
AI	0.18	0.57	1.5	1.9	2.3	2.3	2.3	2.3	2.0	1.8	2.3	2.3	2.3	2.3
UL	ND	ND	2.3	2.9	3.4	3.6	3.6	3.6	3.6	3.6	3.6	3.6	3.6	3.6
Zinc (mg/d)														
EAR	–	2.5	2.5	4.0	7.0	Male 8.5 / Female 7.3	Male 9.4 / Female 6.8	Male 9.4 / Female 6.8	Male 9.4 / Female 6.8	Male 9.4 / Female 6.8	10.5	9.5	10.9	10.4
RDA	–	3	3	5	8	Male 11 / Female 9	Male 11 / Female 8	Male 11 / Female 8	Male 11 / Female 8	Male 11 / Female 8	12	11	13	12
AI	2	–	–	–	–	–	–	–	–	–	–	–	–	–
UL	4	5	7	12	23	34	40	40	40	40	34	40	34	40

RDA = Recommended Dietary Allowance; AI = Adequate Intake; EAR = Estimated Average Requirement; UL = Tolerable Upper Intake Level; ND = Not Determined

Source: Adapted from Otten, *Dietary Reference Intakes: The Essential Guide to Nutrient Requirements*, 2006.

Appendix B
Antioxidants–Dietary Reference Intakes (DRI) 2000

Nutrient	Life Stage Group	RDA/AI* (µgRAE**/d)	EAR/UL* (µgRAE**/d)	Function	Common Food Sources	Adverse Effects (excess intake)	Special Considerations
Vitamin A (No DRIs currently for carotenoids)	0 to 6 months	–/400	–/600	Normal vision	–Dairy	–Liver toxicity	–Alcoholics and those with liver disease, severe protein malnutrition, and hyperlipidemia, are susceptible to excess preformed Vt. A
	7 to 12 months	–/500	–/600	Gene expression	–Fish	–Nausea	
	1 to 3 years	300/–	210/600		–Liver products	–Vomiting	
	4 to 8 years	400/–	275/900	Reproduction	–Vt. A fortified grains, milk, margarine	–Headache	–Pregnant women, infants, children at risk for toxicity from supplements
Males				Embryonic development		–Increased cerebrospinal pressure	
	9 to 13 years	600/–	445/1700		**Carotenoids:**	–Vertigo	**Carotenoids:**
	14 to 18 years	900/–	630/2800	Immune function	–Dark colored fruits and vegetables	–Blurred vision	–β-carotene supplements should only be taken if at risk for vitamin A deficiency
	19 to 30 years	900/–	625/3000			–Bulging fontanel (in infants)	
	31 to 50 years	900/–	625/3000	Growth		–Macular incoordination	
	51 to 70 years	900/–	625/3000			–Birth defects	–Smokers should avoid supplements
	Over 70 years	900/–	625/3000	**Carotenoids:**		–Reduced bone density	–Steam fts./vegs. with 3-5 grams fat to increase bioavailability from food sources
Females				Conversion into vitamin A		–CNS disorders	
	9 to 13 years	600/–	420/1700			**Carotenoids:**	
	14 to 18 years	700/–	485/2800			–Carotenodermia	–Alcohol/some drugs may↓ absorption
	19 to 30 years	700/–	500/3000			–Lycopenodermia	
	31 to 50 years	700/–	500/3000				
	51 to 70 years	700/–	500/3000				
	Over 70 years	700/–	500/3000				
Pregnancy							
	14 to 18 years	750/–	530/2800				
	19 to 50 years	770/–	550/3000				
Lactation							
	14 to 18 years	1200/–	885/2800				
	19 to 50 years	1300/–	900/3000				

Appendix B *(Continued)*

Nutrient	Life Stage Group	RDA/AI* (mg/d)	EAR/UL* (mg/d)	Function	Common Food Sources	Adverse Effects (excess intake)	Special Considerations
Vitamin C	0 to 6 months	–/40	–/ND	Protective antioxidant	–Broccoli	–GI disturbances (diarrhea, nausea, cramping)	–Smokers need an additional 35 mg/d
	7 to 12 months	–/50	–/ND		–Brussel sprouts	–Kidney stones	–Non-smokers exposed to tobacco smoke need to ensure they are meeting RDA for Vt. C.
	1 to 3 years	15/–	13/400	Formation of cartilage and collagen	–Cabbage	–Excess iron absorption	
	4 to 8 years	25/–	22/650		–Cauliflower		
	Males				–Citrus fruits	–Rebound scurvy	
	9 to 13 years	45/–	39/1200	Regulation of iron storage and absorption	–Citrus juices	–Reduced Vt. B_{12} & copper absorption	
	14 to 18 years	75/–	63/1800		–Potatoes		–Coumadin, birth control pills, and frequent aspirin intake
	19 to 30 years	90/–	75/2000		–Spinach	–Erosion dental enamel	
	31 to 50 years	90/–	75/2000	Immune system protection	–Strawberries		–Discontinue Vt. C supplements two weeks before any lab testing
	51 to 70 years	90/–	75/2000		–Tomatoes		
	Over 70 years	90/–	75/2000		–Tomato juice		
	Females				–Food products fortified with Vt. C		
	9 to 13 years	45/–	39/1200				
	14 to 18 years	65/–	56/1800				
	19 to 30 years	75/–	60/2000				
	31 to 50 years	75/–	60/2000				
	51 to 70 years	75/–	60/2000				
	Over 70 years	75/–	60/2000				
	Pregnancy						
	14 to 18 years	80/–	66/1800				
	19 to 50 years	85/–	70/2000				
	Lactation						
	14 to 18 years	115/–	96/1800				
	19 to 50 years	120/–	100/2000				

126

Vitamin E

Age group			Functions	Food sources	Toxicity	Considerations
0 to 6 months	—/4	—/ND	Chain-breaking antioxidant	–Fruits	–Hemorrhagic toxicity	–Patients on anticoagulant therapies should be monitored if taking vitamin E supplements
7 to 12 months	—/5	—/ND		–Meats		–Premature infants
1 to 3 years	6/—	5/200	Strengthens red blood cell membranes	–Nuts		–Head and neck cancer patients
4 to 8 years	7/—	6/300		–Unprocessed cereal grains		–Vitamin K deficiency
Males			Synthesize heme & essential body compounds	–Vegetables		–Fat malabsorption or genetic diseases
9 to 13 years	11/—	9/600		–Vegetable oils		
14 to 18 years	15/—	12/800				
19 to 30 years	15/—	12/1000	Support cellular respiration			
31 to 50 years	15/—	12/1000				
51 to 70 years	15/—	12/1000	Improve vasodilation			
Over 70 years	15/—	12/1000				
Females						
9 to 13 years	11/—	9/600	Inhibit platelet clumping			
14 to 18 years	15/—	12/800				
19 to 30 years	15/—	12/1000				
31 to 50 years	15/—	12/1000				
51 to 70 years	15/—	12/1000				
Over 70 years	15/—	12/1000				
Pregnancy						
14 to 18 years	15/—	12/800				
19 to 50 years	15/—	12/1000				
Lactation						
14 to 18 years	19/—	16/800				
19 to 50 years	19/—	16/1000				

127

Appendix B *(Continued)*

Nutrient	Life Stage Group	RDA/AI* (µg/d)	EAR/UL* (µg/d)	Function	Common Food Sources	Adverse Effects (excess intake)	Special Considerations
Selenium	0 to 6 months	–/15	–/45	Defends against oxidative stress by regulating Vt. C redox	–Cereals & grains –Dairy products –Eggs –Fruits –Muscle meats –Seafood –Vegetables (depending on growing area)	–Hair and nail brittleness –Irritability –Nervous system abnormalities –GI disturbances –Fatigue –Garlic breath odor –Discolored/decayed teeth –Skin rashes	–Vegetarians and those living in low-selenium farming regions may be at risk for deficiency
	7 to 12 months	–/20	–/60				
	1 to 3 years	20/–	17/90				
	4 to 8 years	30/–	23/150				
	Males						
	9 to 13 years	40/–	35/280	Thyroid hormone regulation			
	14 to 18 years	55/–	45/400				
	19 to 30 years	55/–	45/400	Protective effect on red blood cells			
	31 to 50 years	55/–	45/400				
	51 to 70 years	55/–	45/400				
	Over 70 years	55/–	45/400				
	Females			Protects against mercury & cadmium toxicities			
	9 to 13 years	40/–	35/280				
	14 to 18 years	55/–	45/400				
	19 to 30 years	55/–	45/400				
	31 to 50 years	55/–	45/400				
	51 to 70 years	55/–	49/400				
	Over 70 years	55/–	45/400				
	Pregnancy						
	14 to 18 years	60/–	49/400				
	19 to 50 years	60/–	49/400				
	Lactation						
	14 to 18 years	70/–	59/400				
	19 to 50 years	70/–	59/400				

*RDA = Recommended Dietary Allowance; AI = Adequate Intake; EAR = Estimated Average Requirement; UL = Tolerable Upper Intake Level; ND = Not Determined

**RAE = Retinol Activity Equivalent

Source: Adapted from Otten, *Dietary Reference Intakes, The Essential Guide to Nutrient Requirements,* 2006.

Appendix C
Resources

Resource	URL	Comments
Government Sites		
Center for Food Safety and Applied Nutrition, FDA	www.cfsan.fda.gov www.cfsan.fda.gov/~dms/supplmnt.html	Regulatory information about foods and supplements.
Food and Information Center, USDA	www.cnpp.usda.gov	Helpful resource for consumers providing sound nutrition information.
National Center for Complementary and Alternative Medicine, NIH	http://nccam.nih.gov http://nccam.nih.gov/health/bottle http://nccam.nih.gov/health	Provides information about complementary and alternative medicine, including vitamins and minerals.
Office of Dietary Supplements, NIH	http://ods.od.nih.gov http://ods.od.nih.gov/health_Information/Health_Information.aspx http://ods.od.nih.gov/health_Information/IBIDS.aspx	Dietary supplement information and resources; IBIDS database.
PubMed	www.ncbi.nlm.nih.gov/entrez/query.fcgi?DB=pubmed	Provides abstracts from published studies.
U.S. National Library of Medicine, NIH	http://medineplus.gov www.nlm.nih.gov/medlineplus/druginformation.html	Health information on numerous diseases, nutrition topics, and supplements and herbals.
Professional Sites		
Alternative Medicine Foundation	www.amfoundation.org	Evidence based information on alternative medicine.
Arbor Nutrition Guide	www.arborcom.com	Food and nutrition journal abstracts; vitamin/mineral/food information.
Cochrane Systematic Reviews	www.cochrane.org	Provides reviews of studies and offers library sources.
International Food and Information Council	www.ific.org/publications/factsheets/index.cfm	Fact sheets on functional foods and antioxidants.
Natural Medicines Comprehensive Database	www.naturaldatabase.com	Fee-based database of drugs, vitamin, minerals, natural products for safety and efficacy.

(Continued)

Appendix C (*Continued*)

Resource	URL	Comments
U.S. Pharmacopeia	www.usp.org	Official public standards-setting authority for all prescription and over-the-counter medicines, dietary supplements, and other healthcare products manufactured and sold in the United States.
Univ. of Texas at El Paso and Univ. Texas Austin Cooperative Pharmacy Program	www.herbalsafety.utep.edu/	Herbal fact sheets.
University of Maryland Medical Center	www.umm.edu/altmed/index.htm	Fact sheets on supplements and herbs.
Associations		
American Dietetic Association	www.eatright.org	Professional association of nutrition professionals.
Council for Responsible Nutrition	www.crnusa.org	Trade association representing dietary supplement ingredient suppliers and manufacturers—provides a perspective on the industry.
National Natural Foods Association	www.nnfa.org	Trade association that supports the natural products industry—provides a perspective on the industry.
Consumer Friendly Sites		
Almond Board of CA	http://getyoure.com/iu/?mmltemnumber=1487	Vt. E conversion calculator.
CDC	www.fruitsandveggiesmorematters.org	Collaborative effort to increase public consumption of fruits and vegetables; vitamin/mineral information, recipes, and more.
ConsumerLab.com	www.consumerlab.com	Independent test results and information for consumers & healthcare professionals about nutrition products.

130

Appendix C (*Continued*)

Resource	URL	Comments
U.S. Pharmacopeia	www.usp.org	Official public standards-setting authority for all prescription and over-the-counter medicines, dietary supplements, and other healthcare products manufactured and sold in the United States.
Univ. of Texas at El Paso and Univ. Texas Austin Cooperative Pharmacy Program	www.herbalsafety.utep.edu/	Herbal fact sheets.
University of Maryland Medical Center	www.umm.edu/altmed/index.htm	Fact sheets on supplements and herbs.
Associations		
American Dietetic Association	www.eatright.org	Professional association of nutrition professionals.
Council for Responsible Nutrition	www.crnusa.org	Trade association representing dietary supplement ingredient suppliers and manufacturers—provides a perspective on the industry.
National Natural Foods Association	www.nnfa.org	Trade association that supports the natural products industry—provides a perspective on the industry.
Consumer Friendly Sites		
Almond Board of CA	http://getyoure.com/iu/?mnItemnumber=1487	Vt. E conversion calculator.
CDC	www.fruitsandveggiesmorematters.org	Collaborative effort to increase public consumption of fruits and vegetables; vitamin/mineral information, recipes, and more.
ConsumerLab.com	www.consumerlab.com	Independent test results and information for consumers & healthcare professionals about nutrition products.

131

Organization	Website	Description
Executive Office of the President & USDA	www.healthierus.gov	Accurate information to help Americans choose healthier habits.
FDA	www.fda.gov/consumer	Consumer Health Information e-newsletter.
Harvard School of Public Health	www.hsph.harvard.edu/nutritionsource	Resource about diet and nutrition.
HHS & USDA	www.health.gov/dietaryguidelines	"Dietary Guidelines for Americans 2005".
Mayo Clinic	www.mayoclinic.com/health/drug-information/DrugHerbIndex	Information on drugs and supplements.
Memorial Sloan-Kettering Cancer Center	www.mskcc.org/mskcc/html/11570.cfm	Herb, supplement, and botanical information.
National Cancer Institute	www.cancer.gov/cancertopics/treatment/cam http://riskfactor.cancer.gov/DHQ	Information about cancer and CAM therapies; self-administered food questionnaire to evaluate cancer risk.
National Council Against Health Fraud	www.ncahf.com	Private, nonprofit, volunteer agency focusing on health misinformation and fraud with goal to protect the public.
NY Online Access To Health (NOAH)	www.noah-health.org	NY city libraries make easy to understand healthcare information accessible to the layperson; English and Spanish translations provided.
Office of Disease Prevention and Health Promotion, DHHS	www.healthfinder.gov	Collaborative federal website for consumers.
Stephen Barrett, M.D.	www.quackwatch.com	Investigates regulations, medicines, and therapies that are questionable.
The Center for Nutrition Policy and Promotion, USDA	www.mypyramid.gov	Consumer nutrition help site.
USDA	www.fsis.usda.gov/Regulations_&_Policies/Certified_Organic/index.asp	Explains organic food labels.

Note: These resources provide accurate information about vitamins, minerals, dietary supplements, foods, and nutrition topics from reputable and reliable organizations.

GLOSSARY

abetalipoproteinemia: genetic disease that affects the absorption of dietary fats, cholesterol, and vitamins E, A, and sometimes K.

acrodermatitis enteropathica: autosomal recessive zinc deficiency disease characterized by dermatitis, alopecia, and diarrhea.

AI (Adequate Intake): Dietary Reference Intake nutrient value recommended by the IOM for healthy individuals when an RDA cannot be determined.

α-**carotene (alpha carotene):** carotenoid found in food sources.

α-**tocopherol (alpha-tocopherol):** the most biologically active form of vitamin E in humans.

AMDR: Acceptable Macronutrient Distribution Range.

anaerobe: an organism able to survive and function in an environment without oxygen.

anaphylaxis: allergic reaction to a foreign substance after initial exposure.

anoxic: lacking oxygen.

anthocyanins: pigments responsible for the red, blue, and purple colors in fruits and vegetables; possible antioxidant properties.

Anthropoidea: in the biological classification of primates, the haplorrhines, or "dry-nosed" primates, are members of the Haplorrhini clade: the prosimian tarsiers and all true simians (the monkeys and the apes, including humans); Anthropoidea is the former term for the infraorder Simiiformes that includes two parvorders: Platyrrhini (the New World monkeys) and Catarrhini (the Old World monkeys and apes) that split about 40 million years ago (current theory has the ape/monkey split happening in Africa about 25 million years ago); the recent discovery of three new anthropoid fossils in Pakistan's Bugti Hills is causing some scientists to revise this thinking and the classifications of primates may be in for yet another reorganization.

apoptosis: cell death.

arrhythmia: irregular heartbeat.

ascorbic acid, ascorbate: also known as vitamin C; a water-soluble antioxidant vitamin required for the synthesis of collagen and dentin; collagen is the structural component of blood vessels, bones, ligaments, and tendons, while dentin is the structural component of teeth; vitamin C is also an effective antioxidant that protects proteins and genetic materials (RNA and DNA) from damage by free radicals and recycles other oxidized antioxidants, such as vitamin E.

ataxia: inability to control muscles.

atherogenic: formation of fatty deposits in blood vessel arteries.

ATP (Adenosine triphosphate): important carrier of energy in body cells and a compound important in the synthesis of RNA; it is a nucleotide and produced as needed by the body from foods.

autoimmune diseases: diseases that result when the body is attacked by its immune system; genetics plays a major factor in development and includes arthritis, thyroid disease, and diabetes.

Ayurveda: massage technique that claims to improve circulation and remove toxins from the body.

beri-beri: vitamin deficiency disease in which the body does not have adequate thiamine (vitamin B_1) levels. Caused by either poor diet, alcohol abuse, or a rare genetic disease.

β-carotene (beta carotene): provitamin A carotenoid found in food sources; converted into vitamin A when body stores are low.

β-cryptoxanthin (beta-cryptoxanthin): provitamin A carotenoid found in food sources; converted into vitamin A when body stores are low.

bioavailability: measure of how much of a nutrient is absorbed by the body from a given source.

bioflavonoids: term synonymous with flavonoid and refers to a class of polyphenolic plant secondary metabolites found in particularly high concentrations in fruits and vegetables. Flavonoids are most commonly known for their antioxidant activity; however, flavonoid health benefits in cancer and heart disease result from mechanisms other than antioxidant mechanisms.

biomolecules: organic molecule biosynthesized by living organisms (i.e., nucleic acid, protein).

bis-allylic position: the position of the hydrogen adjacent to a double bond in the chemical structure of the fatty acid.

botanicals: component of a plant (herb, fruit, or vegetable) that has been shown to have some nutritional benefit.

bronchodilators: medication that improves the ability to breath.

CAM: complementary and alternative medicine therapies.

Carboniferous era: a geological period of time on Earth, approximately 360 million to 286 million years ago, characterized geologically by rich deposits of coal.

cardiomyopathy: group of diseases that affect the myocardium (muscle of the heart). There are three basic types of cardiomyopathy: dilated cardiomyopathy, hypertrophic cardiomyopathy, and restrictive cardiomyopathy, all of which lead to serious heart malfunction.

CARET (Carotene and Retinol Efficacy Trial): NCI funded study investigating the benefit of combining β-carotene and vitamin A (retinol) supplements to prevent lung and other cancers.

carnitine: amino acid found in nearly all cells of the body; plays a critical role in energy production.

carotenodermia: non-life-threatening yellow discoloration of the skin resulting from overconsumption (30 mg/day or more over long periods of time) of β-carotene.

carotenoids: pigments occurring naturally in plants and thought to have antioxidant properties.

catalyst: substance that enables a chemical reaction to proceed more quickly or under different circumstances than usual.

catechins: polyphenolic antioxidant plant metabolites, specifically flavonoids called flavan-3-ols. Although present in numerous plant species, the largest source in the human diet is from various teas derived from the tea-plant Camellia sinensis; purported to be potent antioxidants.

CDC (The Centers for Disease Control and Prevention): one of the operating branches of the Department of Health and Human Services that promotes health and quality of life by preventing and controlling disability, injury, and disease.

celiac sprue: digestive disease that damages the small intestine and impairs the ability to tolerate gluten found in wheat, rye, and barley and absorb nutrients from foods.

chlorophyll: green pigment in the photosystem elements of chloroplasts that helps plants obtain energy from light; chlorophyll is crucial for photosynthesis.

Co-enzyme Q10 (also known as ubiquinone, ubidecarenone, or CoQ10): is a benzoquinone found in mitochondria of all human cells and is a cofactor in the mitochondrial electron transport chain. CoQ10 in its reduced form (ubiquinol) is also an important antioxidant in both mitochondria and lipid membranes.

collagen: main protein of connective tissue in animals

Commission on the Nomenclature of Inorganic Chemistry: a commission of the International Union of Pure and Applied Chemistry charged with the responsibility for providing nomenclature to the chemical community and whose Rules for Inorganic Nomenclature were published and revised in 1958 and 1970.

cosmoceuticals: cosmetics to which food extracts or ingredients are added.

covalent: chemical bond formed between atoms by the sharing of electrons.

Crohn's disease: inflammatory bowel disease that is often genetic.

cyanobacteria: photosynthetic bacteria usually blue-green in color; also called blue-green algae.

cystic fibrosis: hereditary disease of the exocrine glands characterized by abnormal production of viscous secretions.

cytochrome oxidase multi-protein assembly complex: The enzyme cytochrome c oxidase or Complex IV (PDB 2OCC, EC 1.9.3.1); a large transmembrane protein complex found in bacteria and the mitochondrion; the last protein in the electron transport chain; receives an electron from each of four cytochrome c molecules, and transfers them to one oxygen molecule, converting molecular oxygen to two molecules of water. In the process, it translocates four protons, helping to establish a chemiosmotic potential that the ATP synthase then uses to synthesize ATP.

cytosol: synonymous with cytoplasm, which also includes the organelles; is the internal fluid of the cell.

DHKS: Diet and Health Knowledge Survey.

Dietary Standard for Canada: daily nutrient recommendations for healthy Canadian population.

dioxygen (O_2): most common molecular form of the chemical element oxygen under normal conditions. It constitutes about 20 percent of atmospheric air, is the essential agent in the respiration of plants and animals, and is necessary to support combustion.

dismutation: a chemical reaction in which an element is simultaneously reduced and oxidized to form two different products.

DNA: deoxyribonucleic acid; molecule that contains the genetic instructions for all living organisms.

dopamine: neurotransmitter that transmits signals between nerve cells.

DRI (Dietary Reference Intakes): recommended daily nutrient intakes for all healthy Americans established by the IOM.

DSHEA: Dietary Supplement Health and Education Act of 1994; loosened tight control by the FDA over dietary supplements sold to consumers.

Dumas, Jean Baptiste Andre′ (1800–1884): discovered that food possessed other important nutrients beside carbohydrates, proteins, and fats.

EAR (Estimated Average Requirement): DRI recommended by the IOM that meets the requirements of half of the healthy individuals in a specific age or gender group.

ecchymoses: (also known as a bruise or contusion) a kind of injury to biological tissue in which the capillaries are damaged, allowing blood to seep into the surrounding tissue.

EGCG: epigallocatechin-3-gallate; a polyphenolic phytochemical found in tea.

electrons: elementary particle with a negative charge.

endogenous: originating or produced within an organism, tissue, or cell.

ephedra, ephedrine, ephedrine alkaloids: derivatives of ma huang, a naturally occurring plant amine used in Chinese medicine for thousands of years for cold and asthma symptoms. The alkaloids ephedrine and pseudoephedrine are the primary active ingredients used in OTC bronchodilators and decongestant medicines; the center of controversy in the United States after widespread use in dietary supplements resulted in numerous adverse events and death.

epicatechin: a flavonoid in the polyphenol classification.

erythropoietic protoporphyria: inherited enzyme deficiency in which the skin is overly sensitive to sun exposure.

eukaryotes: organisms (including animals, plants, fungi, and protists) with a complex cell or cells, where the genetic material is organized into a membrane-bound nucleus or nuclei. Eukaryotic cells also contain membrane-bound organelles such as mitochondria and chloroplasts. Eukaryotes are differentiated from prokaryotes (bacteria and archaea) that lack membrane-bound organelles and other complex cell structures.

exogenous: originating or produced outside of the body.

fat-soluble: nutrient that requires the presence of fat to facilitate absorption by the body.

FD&C Act: Federal Food, Drug, and Cosmetic Act.

FDA: U.S. Food and Drug Administration.

Fe^{2+}: ferrous iron.

Fenton reaction: a chemical reaction, which is the iron-salt-dependent decomposition of dihydrogen peroxide that generates the highly reactive and biologically dangerous hydroxyl radical.

flavonoids: a large class of polyphenolic plant secondary metabolites found in particularly high concentrations in fruits and vegetables. Flavonoids are excellent antioxidants in vitro and have significant effects on enzymes and signal transduction mechanism in plant and animal cells.

folate, folic acid, folacin: folate (also called folacin) is the biologically active form of vitamin B; necessary for red blood cell production; folic acid refers to the synthetic form used in supplements.

Food Additives Amendment: legislation of 1958 that regulated all substances added to food as a public safety measure.

Free radicals: highly reactive molecules that lack paired electrons and that can oxidize other molecules and cause cell tissue damage.

Free radical theory of aging: theory proposed by Denham Harmon that suggests consequences of aging result from attacks by radicals generated primarily in the cell mitochondria during normal metabolism.

French Paradox: a name for the perceived paradox that people in France suffer relatively low incidence of coronary heart disease, despite their diet allegedly being rich in saturated fats. The term is often confused with the related but different notion of the Mediterranean diet.

frugivores: mammals that eat fruits.

functional food: any food or food ingredient that may provide a health benefit beyond the traditional nutrients it contains.

Funk, Casimir: anglicized from Kazimierz, a Polish biochemist; credited with developing the concept of vitamins in 1912, which he called vital amines or vitamines.

g/gm: gram; a metric unit of measure.

gallic acid: a simple organic phenolic acid found widely in plants or combined with plant tannins. Gallic acid is chemically known as 3,4,5-trihydroxybenzoic acid and is in high concentration in gallnuts, hence the name. It is commonly used as a standard reference compound when measuring phenolic compounds in plants and foods.

γ-tocopherol (gamma-tocopherol): one of four different forms or isomers of tocopherol.

GMP (Good Manufacturing Practice Regulations): standardized production regulations for drugs and foods to prevent errors causing consumer harm.

GPx: glutathione peroxidases.

GPx1, GPx2, GPx3, GPx4: glutathione peroxidases; selenoproteins that defend against oxidative stresses.

GRAS (Generally Recognized As Safe): ingredients that are known to be safe to add to foods.

GSH (gamma-glutamyl-cysteinyl-glycine): the tripeptide glutathione (GSH) containing an unusual peptide linkage between the amine group of cysteine and the carboxyl group of the glutamate side chain. Glutathione, an antioxidant, protects cells from toxins such as free radicals.

GSSG: oxidized glutathione, also known as glutathione disulphide.

gulonolactone oxidase: L-gulonolactone oxidase (EC 1.1.3.8); an enzyme that catalyzes the reaction of D-glucuronolactone (also known as L-gulono-1, 4-lactone) with oxygen to produce L-xylo-hex-3-ulonolactone and hydrogen peroxide; uses FAD (flavin–adenine dinucleotide) as a cofactor.

H. pylori (helicobacter pylori): bacteria believed responsible for most peptic ulcer disease.

Haber-Weiss reaction: oxidized glutathione, also known as glutathione disulphide.

haem: a prosthetic group that consists of an iron atom contained in the center of a large heterocyclic porphyrin. Porphyrin-containing metalloproteins can contain other metals, but if they contain iron they are known as hemoproteins.

Harman, Denham: scientist who proposed the "free radical theory of aging."

heme: synonymous with haem (see above).

hemochromatosis: iron overload; when the body stores excess iron in body tissues leading to disease.

hemolytic anemia: blood disorder in which red blood cells are destroyed.

hemorrhage: profuse bleeding.

hepatic: acting on or occurring in the liver.

Herodotus: Greek historian (484–425 B.C.); one of the first to observe and write about the connection between sunshine upon the skin and improved durability of the bones.

HHANES: Hispanic Health and Nutrition Examination Survey.

Hippocrates: considered the "Father of Medicine"; made the connection between diet and health.

hydrogen peroxide: weak acid that has strong oxidizing properties especially in biological systems.

hydroxyl radicals: chemical structure $OH^\bullet$; is the neutral form of the hydroxide ion and highly reactive and consequently short lived. An important part of radical chemistry, hydroxyl radicals are produced from the decomposition of hydro-peroxides (ROOH) or by the reaction of excited atomic oxygen with water.

hydroxylase: group of enzymes that catalyze the formation of a hydroxyl group on a substrate by incorporation of one atom (monooxygenases) or two atoms (dioxygenases) of oxygen from O_2.

hydroxylation: chemical interaction that oxidizes a compound by adding one or more hydroxyl (–OH) groups.

hyperkeratosis: thickening of the outer layer of the skin.

hyperlipidemia: elevation of lipids in the bloodstream that cause heart disease.

hypernutrition: excess nutrient intakes.

hypervitaminosis: negative health effects caused by excess intake of one or more vitamins.

hypoxia: shortage of oxygen in the body.

IFIC: International Information Council Foundation.

in situ: Latin for in the original position.

in vitro: New Latin for in glass or in an artificial environment outside the living organism.

in vivo: Latin for within a living organism.

iodothyronine deiodinases: (EC 1.97.1.10) is an enzyme important in the action of thyroid hormones and is an unusual selenoprotein as it contains a rare amino acid selenocysteine.

IOM: Institute of Medicine of the National Academies.

ion: atom or group of atoms that have lost or gained one or more electrons, changing their charge.

ionizing: converting an atom or molecule into an ion by changing the difference between the number of protons and electrons.

iron: a chemical element with the symbol Fe that is both an essential and a toxic mineral in biology; integrated into many proteins and enzymes, but it can enter potentially destructive reactions if not carefully chaperoned by molecules like transferrin.

isoflavone: a class of organic compounds and biomolecules related to the flavonoids that act as phytoestrogens in mammals. They are found in high concentrations in soy beans.

IU (international unit): quantity of a biologically active substance, such as a vitamin or hormone; accepted as an international standard.

IUPAC (International Union of Pure and Applied Chemistry): an international nongovernmental organization established in 1919 devoted to the advancement of chemistry and includes national chemistry societies as members. It is the recognized authority in developing standards for the naming of the chemical elements and their compounds, through its Interdivisional Committee on Nomenclature and Symbols (IUPAC nomenclature). It is a member of the International Council for Science (ICSU).

joint effusion: abnormal build up of fluid in the joints; usually associated with arthritis.

Kashin-Beck disease: endemic disease of the cartilage that usually occurs in preadolescents or adolescents living in low-selenium farm areas.

Keshan disease: occurs in selenium-deficient children under stress (such as an infection) and causes cardiomyopathy.

kwashiorkor: malnutrition caused by inadequate protein intake despite adequate intakes of total calories.

Lavoisier, Antoine: considered the Father of Nutrition; became the first scientist to document the interrelationship between food and energy metabolism in the body.

LDL: low-density lipoprotein; a complex of lipids and proteins, with greater amounts of lipid than protein, that transports cholesterol in the blood. High levels are associated with an increased risk of atherosclerosis and coronary heart disease.

legume: a plant in the family Fabaceae (or Leguminosae), or a fruit of these plants. Well-known legumes include alfalfa, clover, peas, beans, lentils, lupins, and peanuts. Legume plants are renowned for their ability to fix atmospheric nitrogen and hence naturally fertilize soils. This ability stems from a symbiotic relationship with certain bacteria known as rhizobia found in legume root nodules.

lignin: a chemical compound (complex, highly cross-linked aromatic polymer) that is most commonly derived from wood and is an integral part of the cell walls of plants; one of most abundant organic compounds on earth after cellulose and chitin.

Lind, James: physician for the British Navy who carried out the first controlled nutrition experiment and "discovered" the cure for scurvy in 1747.

lipid: organic fat molecule that is insoluble in water; cholesterol molecule is one example; used for energy storage and serves as structural components in cell membranes.

lipid peroxidation: oxidative breakdown of lipids.

lipoprotein: biochemical molecule that contains both proteins and lipids.

lutein: A yellow carotenoid pigment found widely in nature; it is a xanthophyll and is a nonprovitamin carotenoid that cannot be converted into vitamin A.

lycopene: a red pigment found in high concentrations in tomatoes and palm oils. Lycopene is considered chemically to be the parent substance from which all natural carotenoid pigments are derived. It cannot however be converted into vitamin A in humans.

lycopenodermia: a deep orange skin discoloration that results from excess lycopene intake.

lysine hydroxylases: enzyme responsible for hydroxylation of lysine.

ma huang: cone bearing shrub native to China that is used to make ephedra alkaloids for medicinal use.

macronutrients: nutrients that provide energy to an organism: carbohydrate, protein, fat.

macrophage respiratory burst (oxidative burst): the rapid release of reactive oxygen species (superoxide radical and hydrogen peroxide) from different types of cells, especially the macrophage. These chemicals are released as a function of immune cells, e.g. neutrophils and macrophages, as they come into contact with different bacteria or fungi. Respiratory burst plays an important role in the immune system. It is a crucial reaction that occurs in phagocytes to degrade internalized particles and bacteria. Within the immune cell, NADPH oxidase produces superoxide, spontaneously recombines with other molecules to produce reactive free radicals. Myeloperoxidase uses one of these free radicals, hydrogen peroxide, to produce hypochlorous acid that is lethal to invading organisms.

malnutrition: a condition of poor nutrition because of an insufficient or poorly balanced diet or faulty digestion or utilization of foods.

McCollum, Elmer Vernon: research scientist who conducted numerous nutrition studies in the 1920s; credited with discovering vitamins A and B and demonstrating the importance of vitamin D, calcium, phosphorus, fluorine, magnesium, manganese, iron, zinc, sodium, potassium, boron, and cobalt.

MedWatch: FDA safety information and adverse event reporting program.

Menke's disease: disease caused by a defective gene that regulates copper metabolism in the body.

μg: micrograms; unit of metric measurement.

mg: milligram; a metric unit of mass equal to one thousandth (10^{-3}) of a gram.

micronutrients: essential elements needed in small amounts for good health, for example, vitamins and minerals.

mitochondria: organelles in most eukaryotes found outside the nucleus, which produces energy for cells through cellular respiration. Mitochondria, as the principal sites of ATP synthesis, contain enzymes of the tricarboxylic acid cycle and for fatty acid oxidation, oxidative phosphorylation, and many other biochemical pathways. They contain their own nucleic acids and ribosomes, replicate independently, and code for the synthesis of some of their own proteins mitochondria.

mitochondrial encephalomyopathies: diseases that affect the nervous system and/or skeletal muscles and are caused by genetic abnormalities in the mitochondria.

National Academy of Sciences: agency that brings together scientific and technological experts to address critical national issues and provide advice to the federal government and public.

NCCAM: the National Center for Complementary and Alternative Medicine; is one of the twenty-seven institutes and centers that make up the National Institutes of Health (NIH) within the Department of Health and Human Services of the federal government of the United States.

NCHS: National Center for Health Statistics.

NCI: National Cancer Institute; part of the United States Federal government's National Institutes of Health.

neural tube: developing vertebrate nervous system.

neurodegenerative diseases: incurable disease caused by gradual loss of neurons, eventually leading to death, e.g. Alzheimer's.

neurotransmitter: chemicals used to relay and amplify signals between neurons and other cells.

neurotransmitters: a substance that transmits nerve impulses across a synapse.

neutron: uncharged elementary particle.

NFCS: National Food Consumption Survey.

NHANES (Health and Nutrition Examination Survey): one of the most comprehensive and objective national surveys that studies a representative sample of the U.S. population using direct interview, physical examination, and medical record reviews analyzing health, lifestyle, and diet.

NHIS: National Health Interview Survey.

NIH: National Institutes of Health; is a federally funded research and development center composed of eight agencies that compose the Public Health Service in the United States Department of Health and Human Services.

NMI: National Marketing Institute.

NNFA: National Nutritional Foods Association.

nonheme iron: form of iron that is not well absorbed by the body.

nonprovitamin A carotenoids: carotenoids that cannot be converted to vitamin A in the body, for example, lycopene, lutein, and zeaxanthin.

noradrenaline: neurotransmitter released by nerve cells.

nucleic acid: a high-molecular-weight nucleotide polymer that include deoxyribonucleic acid (DNA) and ribonucleic acid (RNA).

nucleotide: the central core of a body or object; in the case of a cell it is a spheroid body consisting of a thin nuclear membrane, with one or more nucleoli, chromatin, linin, and nucleoplasm. The organelle carries the genetic information for eukaryotic cells.

nucleus: cell organelle of eukaryotes essential to cell functions.

nutraceuticals: category of functional foods, cosmoceuticals, and dietary supplements that possess (in theory) disease-preventive qualities.

Nutrient Databank System: data on composition of foods maintained by the USDA.

nutrigenomics: the application of the sciences of genomics, transcriptomics, proteomics, and metabolomics to human nutrition, especially the relationship between nutrition and health.

ODS: The Office of Dietary Supplements; is part of the NIH charged with the mission of promoting scientific research in the area of dietary supplements.

OTC: over-the-counter.

oxidase: any enzyme of the class of oxidoreductases in which molecular oxygen is the hydrogen acceptor. These are enzymes that catalyze an oxidation/reduction reaction.

oxidation: the combination of a substance with oxygen or a reaction in which the atoms in an element lose electrons.

oxidative stress: imbalance between the production of reactive oxygen or reactive nitrogen species and the ability to control these radicals or repair the damage they do to important biomolecules.

oxygenase: enzyme that transfers oxygen to a substrate.

Paleozoic era: period of time on Earth approximately 543 to 248 million years ago.

pellagra: disease that results from a niacin deficiency.

peripheral neuropathy: damage to the peripheral nervous system.

Permian-Triassic transition: period of time on Earth approximately 250 million years ago; during the last period of the Palaeozoic Era, many species became extinct. The Permian-Triassic extinction event was the most extensive extinction event recorded in paleontology with 90 to 95 percent of marine species becoming extinct, as well as 70 percent of all land organisms.

peroxidases: peroxidases (EC number 1.11.1.x) are a large family of enzymes that catalyze the reaction: $ROOR' + $ electron donor $(2\ e-) + 2H+ \rightarrow ROH + R'OH$. The optimal substrate of many of these enzymes is hydrogen peroxide, but some use organic hydroperoxides such as lipid peroxides as their substrates. Peroxidases can contain a heme cofactor in their active sites, or redox-active cysteine or selenocysteine residues.

peroxyl radicals: an intermediate product of lipid peroxidation (or the oxidative degradation of lipids). When free radicals take electrons from lipids in cell membranes, free radicals of lipids are produced leading to an oxidative chain reaction mechanism. It most often affects polyunsaturated fatty acids, because they contain multiple double bonds in between which lie methylene $-CH2-$ groups that possess especially reactive hydrogens. When a lipid radical reacts with another unsaturated lipid molecule a lipid peroxyl radical is produced.

petechiae: red or purplish spots that appear on the skin from local hemorrhaging.

Phase 1 enzymatic processes: metabolic processes that represent the biochemical l modification or degradation of toxic or xenobiotic molecules in the body, usually through specialized enzymatic systems. During xenobiotic metabolism lipophilic chemical compounds are often converted into more readily excreted polar products. The process is divided into two parts: Phase 1 and Phase 2. Phase I reactions usually precedes Phase II, though not necessarily. Phase I reactions (also termed nonsynthetic reactions) may occur by oxidation, reduction, hydrolysis, cyclization, and decyclization reactions. The process of oxidation usually involves mixed function oxidases and mono-oxygenases in the liver and typically involve a cytochrome p-450 haemoprotein, NADPH and oxygen. Many phase I products require further metabolism to produce a highly polar conjugate for efficient elimination from the body (Phase 2 reactions).

Phase 2 enzymatic processes: a continuation of the Phase 1 reaction of xenobiotic metabolism and known as conjugation reactions (e.g., with glucuronic acid, sulfonates [commonly known as sulfation], glutathione or amino acids). These reactions are effective in detoxification of many toxic products of Phase 1 metabolism and they also render phase I metabolites more hydrophilic and thus more easily removed from the body (see Phase 1 reactions).

phenol: hydroxyl derivatives of aromatic hydrocarbons.

phosphorylation: the combining of a compound with phosphoric acid or a phosphorus containing group.

photosynthesis: formation of energy in plant cells from carbon dioxide and hydrogen when plants are exposed to light.

photosystem PSII: protein complexes involved in photosynthesis found in photosynthetic membranes of plants, algae and cyanobacteria, or in the cytoplasmic membrane of photosynthetic bacteria. The enzymes of photosystems complexes uses light energy to reduce molecules. Two families of photosystems exist: type I reaction centers (like photosystem I [P700] in chloroplasts and in green-sulphur bacteria) and type II reaction centers (like photosystem II [P680] in chloroplasts and in non-sulphur purple bacteria). The "P" designation refers to the wavelength of light for which the photosystem is most reactive (700 and 680 nanometers, respectively for PSI and PSII in chloroplasts). Type I photosystems use ferredoxin-like iron-sulfur cluster proteins as terminal electron acceptors, while type II photosystems ultimately shuttle electrons to a quinone terminal electron acceptor. Both photosystems form a unique photosynthetic chain in chloroplasts and cyanobacteria that is capable of extracting electrons from water and producing oxygen as a byproduct of the process.

phytates: main storage form of phosphorus in plant cells.

phytochemicals: compounds not found in the body that occur naturally in fruits and vegetables and have a beneficial effect on health.

picolinate (picolinic acid): an isomer of niacin, also known as **nicotinic acid** or **vitamin B$_3$** and a water-soluble vitamin, whose derivatives such as NADH, NAD, NAD$^+$, and NADP play essential roles in energy metabolism in the living cell and DNA repair.

Poison Squad: a group of young men who served as human guinea pigs and agreed to eat only foods that had been treated with measured amounts of chemical preservatives to test the safety and side effects of food preservatives in the early 1900s.

polyploidization: the process by which some biological cells and organisms acquire the presence of more than two homologous sets of chromosomes.

proline hydroxylases: hydrolases are enzymes that catalyze the hydrolysis of a chemical bond. A typical reaction is: $A-B + H_2O \rightarrow A-OH + B-H$. The P class or praline hydrolases catalyze the nucleophilic attack on C1 atom of deoxyribose by uncharged amino group of terminal proline residue (P). Oxidized base of damaged DNA is released and the covalent intermediate is formed. The intermediate (Schiff base) rearranges and decomposes to release 3′-phosphate and the 5′-phosphate and is similarly cleaved.

pro-oxidant: a compound that produces oxygen by-products from normal cell metabolism that can cause damage to cells.

Prosimii: early classification scheme broke the Primate order into the suborders Prosimii (prosimians) and Anthropoidea (simians—monkeys and apes). However the prosimian tarsiers have been shown to be more closely related to the simians, and so it has been moved into the Anthropoidea, which is now renamed as Haplorrhini, and Prosimii renamed as Strepsirrhini.

prospective cohort studies: studies that follow a group of individuals over time looking for health outcomes related to prior information collected.

Proteomics: study of the structure and function of proteins.

Proterozoic period: period of time on Earth, approximately 2.5 billion to 543 million years ago, when banded iron formations were formed and the Earth's atmosphere started to become oxygenic.

Protist: diverse group of eukaryote organisms that cannot be classified in any of the other kingdoms as fungi, animals, or plant; relatively simple organisms, either unicellular, or multicellular without highly specialized tissues.

protons: elementary particle that carries a positive electrical charge.

provitamin A carotenoids: carotenoids that can be converted to vitamin A in the body, for example, α-carotene, β-carotene, and β-cryptoxanthin.

Proxmire bill: 1976 legislation that prohibited the FDA from regulating vitamins and minerals as prescription drugs.

pseudoephedrine: isomer of ephedrine used in nasal decongestants.

PUFA: polyunsaturated fatty acids.

The Pure Food and Drug Act: law that gave the federal government broad authority to protect the public from adulterated and mislabeled drugs and foods.

quench: to put out or bring to an end.

RDA (Recommended Dietary Allowance): DRI recommended by the IOM; daily average nutrient intake for healthy populations that meet daily nutrient requirements.

rebound scurvy: symptoms of scurvy that develop when return to normal dietary intakes of vitamin C after taking megadoses of it.

redox: shorthand for oxidation/reduction reaction.

redox biology: describes all chemical reactions in biological systems in which atoms have their oxidation number (oxidation state) changed. The term redox comes from the two concepts of reduction and oxidation. In simple terms: oxidation describes the loss of electrons by a molecule, atom, or ion. Reduction describes the gain of electrons by a molecule, atom, or ion.

resveratrol: polyphenol and stilbene compound found in red wine, grapes, peanuts, and other plant foods; thought to have antioxidant properties.

retinal: also known as retinaldehyde; is a light-sensitive molecule in the photoreceptor cells of the retina. Retinal is the fundamental chromophore involved in the transduction of light into visual signals, that is, nerve impulses to be sent to the brain.

retinol: the animal form of vitamin A; is a fat-soluble retinoid, antioxidant vitamin important in vision and bone growth. Retinol precursors are ingested from animal sources as retinyl esters and as provitamin A carotenoids. Provitamin A carotenoids are cleaved to produce retinal that is reversibly reduced to produce retinol.

retinopathy: a general term that refers to noninflammatory disorders of the retina that can cause blindness.

retrospective studies: scientific study that looks back at past behaviors.

rickets: bone deformities that are caused by a vitamin D deficiency.

RNI (Recommended Nutrient Intake): establishes daily nutrient standards for Americans; established by the IOM.

RNS: reactive nitrogen species.

ROS: reactive oxygen species.

scurvy: a disease due to deficiency of ascorbic acid (vitamin C), marked by anemia, spongy gums, a tendency to mucocutaneous hemorrhages, and hardening of calf and leg muscles.

selenate, selenite: selenate is an ion, $SeO_4{}^{2-}$; a good oxidizer that can be reduced to selenite ($SeO_3{}^{2-}$) or selenium (Se).

selenide: reduced form of selenium; all forms of selenium are eventually metabolized to this form.

selenium: a chemical nonmetal element, Se, that is chemically related to sulfur. Although it is toxic in large doses, selenium is an essential micronutrient in all known forms of life. It is a component of the unusual amino acids selenocysteine and selenomethionine. In humans, selenium is a trace element nutrient that functions as cofactor for reduction of antioxidant enzymes such as glutathione peroxidases and thioredoxin reductase. It also a cofactor for thyroid hormone deiodinases important to proper thyroid function.

selenocysteine: unusual amino acid that is present in redox; important selenoprotein enzymes are glutathione peroxidases, tetraiodothyronine 5' deiodinases, thioredoxin reductases. Selenocysteine has a structure similar to cysteine, but with an atom of selenium taking the place of the usual sulfur.

selenomethionine: is an amino acid containing selenium and is a common natural food source of selenium. It can not be synthesized by higher animals, but can be obtained from plant material.

selenophosphate synthetase: selenoprotein involved in selenium metabolism.

selenoproteins: is any protein that includes a selenocysteine residue. Selenoproteins exist in all major forms of life, eukaryote, eubacteria, and archaea. Among eukaryotes, selenoproteins appear to be common in animals. Well-known selenoproteins include the glutathione peroxidases that are imposting to antioxidant defenses.

sequester: to remove, set apart, isolate.

Sinclair, Upton: authored *The Jungle*, which exposed the unsanitary meat industry conditions in 1906 and led to food adulteration laws.

singlet oxygen (O_2): the lowest excited state of the dioxygen molecule; occurs when ground state oxygen or triplet oxygen (air) absorbs enough energy to reverse the spin of one of its unpaired electrons; can be highly reactive.

SOD (Cu-Zn-SOD or Mn SOD): one of several common forms of the enzyme superoxide dismutase (SOD, EC 1.15.1.1). SOD's are proteins cofactored with copper and zinc, or manganese, iron, or nickel that catalyzes the dismutation of superoxide into oxygen and hydrogen peroxide. As such, it is an important antioxidant defense in nearly all cells exposed to oxygen. The cytosols of virtually all eukaryotic cells contain an SOD enzyme with copper and zinc (Cu-Zn-SOD).

stilbene: compound formed in trees that may have polyphenolic antioxidant properties. An example of a stilbenoid is reservatrol, which is found in grapes and has been suggested to have many health benefits.

subarachnoid hemorrhage: occurs when the area surrounding the brain fills with blood from a ruptured blood vessel and death results; also called cerebral aneurysm.

substrate: molecule that is acted upon by an enzyme; also the natural living environment of an organism.

superoxide radical: highly reactive oxygen radical formed by a single electron reduction reaction that occurs during normal cell metabolism; capable of devastating cell damage.

tannin: phenolic substance found in plants.

tetrahydrofolic acid: a folic acid derivative produced by dihydrofolate reductase and a coenzyme in many reactions, especially in the metabolism of amino acids and nucleic acids. It acts as a donor of a group with one carbon atom. It gets this carbon atom by sequestering formaldehyde produced in other processes.

thalassemia: genetic blood disorder.

thalidomide: drug used in the 1950s and 1960s in Europe and given to pregnant women for morning sickness in Europe; inadequate safety testing of this drug resulted in thousands of deformed babies being born and more strict drug regulations in the United States.

thiol: compound composed of a sulfur and a hydrogen atom.

thioredoxin: proteins that act as antioxidants by reducing the cysteine thiol-disulfide exchange; found in nearly all organisms and essential for life in mammals.

thioredoxin reductase: selenoprotein that regenerates vitamin C from oxidized metabolites.

tocol: refers to vitamin E compounds having a similar structure incorporating a saturated "tail". Vitamin E, the major fat-soluble antioxidant vitamin, occurs naturally as eight compounds. Four of these compounds have a tocol structure with a saturated C16 phytyl side-chain, and four have a tocotrienol structure with the phytyl side-chain having three double bonds. The term is sometimes used to refer to all forms of tocopherol.

tocopherol: vitamin E, a fat-soluble vitamin in eight forms that is an important antioxidant; often used in skin creams and lotions because it is claimed by the manufacturers to play a role in encouraging skin healing and reducing scarring after injuries such as burns. Natural vitamin E exists in eight different forms or isomers, four tocopherols and four tocotrienols. All isomers have a chromanol ring, with a hydroxyl group that can donate a hydrogen atom to reduce free radicals and a hydrophobic side chain that allows for penetration into biological membranes. There is an alpha, beta, gamma, and delta form of both the tocopherols and tocotrienols, determined by the number of methyl groups on the chromanol ring. Each form has its own biological activity, the measure of potency or functional use in the body.

tryptophan: essential amino acid found in meat sources.

ubiquinone (Co-enzyme Q10): fat-soluble, vitamin-like compound synthesized in cell mitochondria and also found in foods; used as a coenzyme in cell energy production and theorized to scavenge free radicals and improve heart function.

UL (Tolerable Upper Intake Level): DRI recommended by the IOM that is the highest average daily nutrient intake that most likely does not pose a health risk.

urate: salt derived from uric acid when the body cannot metabolize it.

USDA: United States Department of Agriculture.

vasodilation: when blood vessel walls relax and dilate.

Vitamin A: essential fat-soluble vitamin needed for vision, growth, reproduction, and immunity.

Vitamin B: eight essential water-soluble vitamins important in cell metabolism.

Vitamin C (ascorbic acid): essential water-soluble vitamin for all humans; functions as an antioxidant and cofactor in enzyme and hormonal reactions.

Vitamin D: essential fat-soluble vitamin made by the body when exposed to sunlight (UV rays); maintains normal blood levels of calcium and phosphorus; helps to form and maintain strong bones.

Vitamin E (α-tocopherol): essential fat-soluble vitamin that strengthens red blood cell membranes, acts as a chain-breaking antioxidant, synthesizes heme and essential body compounds, and supports cellular respiration.

Vitamin K: essential fat-soluble vitamin required for blood clotting.

Vitamin P: first name given to bioflavonoids.

vitamin precursors: also known as provitamins; cannot be used until converted by the body to its active form.

vitamines: name first given to vitamins by Casimir Funk.

water-soluble: dissolves in a solvent (usually water).

WHO: World Health Organization.

Wiley, Dr. Harvey: head of the Bureau of Chemistry, which is now the FDA.

WPHS: Women's Physicians' Health Study.

xanthine oxidase: XO, (bovine milk enzyme is PDB 1FIQ, EC 1.17.3.2) catalyzes the oxidation of hypoxanthine to xanthine and can further catalyze the oxidation of xanthine to uric acid: hypoxanthine $+ O_2 + H_2O \leftrightarrow$ xanthine $+ H_2O_2$ xanthine $+ O_2 + H_2O \leftrightarrow$ uric acid $+ H_2O_2$

xenobiotic: chemical not normally present in an organism and thus a foreign and sometimes toxic compound.

zeaxanthin: non-provitamin A carotenoid that is one of the two carotenoids contained within the retina. Lutein and zeaxanthin have identical chemical formulas and are isomers, but they are not stereoisomers. The main difference between them is in the location of a double bond in one of the end rings.

zinc: essential micronutrient found in almost every cell.

NOTES

CHAPTER 1

1. National Center for Health Statistics, "Fast Stats A to Z, Life Expectancy," U.S. Department of Health and Human Services, Centers for Disease Control and Prevention, Hyattsville, MD, 2005, http://www.cdc.gov/nchs/fastats/lifexpec.htm (accessed January 4, 2007).

2. National Center for Health Statistics, "Health, United States, 2005 with Chartbook on Trends in the Health of Americans," U.S. Department of Health and Human Services, Centers for Disease Control and Prevention, Hyattsville, MD, 2005, http://www.cdc.gov/nchs/data/hus/hus.05.pdf (accessed January 5, 2007).

3. The Centers for Disease Control and Prevention and the Merck Company Foundation, "The State of Aging and Health in America 2007 Report," U.S. Department of Health and Human Services, Centers for Disease Control and Prevention, Hyattsville, MD, March 2007, http://www.cdc.gov/aging/saha.htm (accessed May 7, 2007).

4. The Centers for Disease Control and Prevention, "The State of Aging and Health," 2007.

5. National Center for Health Statistics, "Health, United States, 2005."

6. Food and Nutrition Board, Board on Life Sciences, Institute of Medicine of the National Academies, *Dietary Supplements: A Framework for Evaluating Safety*, Washington, DC: The National Academies Press, 2005, http://books.nap.edu/openbook. php?record_id=10882&page=R2 (accessed May 15, 2007).

7. "Segment Profile: Vitamins & Minerals," *Nutrition Business Journal* XI, no. 2 (February 2006): 1–11.

8. Charles H. Halsted, "Dietary Supplements and Functional Foods: 2 Sides of a Coin?" *American Journal of Clinical Nutrition* 77, no. 4 (2003): 1001, http://www.ajcn. org/cgi/reprint/77/4/1001S (accessed January 7, 2007).

9. National Institutes of Health, "NIH State-of-the-Science Conference Statement on Multivitamin/Mineral Supplements and Chronic Disease Prevention," *Annals of Internal Medicine* 145 (2006): 364–371, http://consensus.nih.gov/2006/ MVMFINAL080106.pdf (accessed January 12, 2007).

10. I.S. Bass and A.L. Young, "Dietary Supplement Health and Education Act: A Legislative History and Analysis," The Food and Drug Law Institute, Washington, DC,

1996, http://www.fdli.org/pubs/Journal%20Online/50_2/art4.pdf (accessed May 15, 2007).

11. National Center for Health Statistics, "Health United States, 2005."

12. National Center for Health Statistics, "Health, United States, 2006 with Chartbook on Trends in the Health of Americans," U.S. Department of Health and Human Services, Centers for Disease Control and Prevention, Hyattsville, MD, 2006, http://www.cdc.gov/nchs/data/hus/hus.05.pdf (accessed March 4, 2007).

13. Ibid.

14. National Center for Health Statistics, "Health, United States, 2005."

15. Patricia M. Barnes, Eve Powell-Griner, Kim McFann, and Richard Nahin, "Complementary and Alternative Medicine Use among Adults: United States, 2002," *CDC Advance Data from Vital and Health Statistics*, no. 343, May 27, 2004, http://www.cdc.gov/nchs/data/ad/ad343.pdf (accessed May 15, 2007).

16. John A. Astin, Ariane Marie, Kenneth R. Pelletier, Erik Hansen, and William L. Haskell, "A Review of the Incorporation of Complementary and Alternative Medicine by Mainstream Physicians," *Archives of Internal Medicine* 158, no. 21 (1998): 2303–2310, http://archinte.ama-assn.org/cgi/content/full/158/21/2303 (accessed January 15, 2007).

17. The American Dietetic Association Public Relations Team, "Nutrition and You: Trends 2000: What Do Americans Think, Need, Expect?" *Journal of the American Dietetic Association* 100, no. 6 (June 2000): 626–627, http://www.adajournal.org/article/PIIS0002822300001838/fulltext?refuid=PIIS0002822305000659 (accessed January 7, 2007).

18. Sylvia Rowe and Cheryl Toner, "Dietary Supplement Use in Women: The Role of the Media," *The Journal of Nutrition* 133 (2003): 2008S–2009S, http://jn.nutrition.org/cgi/content/full/133/6/2008S (accessed January 8, 2007).

19. Amy E. Millen, Kevin W. Dodd, and Amy F. Subar, "Use of Vitamin, Mineral, Nonvitamin, and Nonmineral Supplements in the United States: The 1987, 1992, and 2000 National Health Interview Survey Results," *Journal of the American Dietetic Association* 104, no. 6 (June 2004): 942–950, http://www.adajournal.org/article/PIIS0002822304004377/fulltext (accessed January 12, 2007).

20. E. R. Miller, R. Pastor-Barriuso, D. Dalal, R. Riemersma, L. J. Appel, and E. Guallar, "Meta-Analysis: High-Dosage Vitamin E Supplementation May Increase All-Cause Mortality," *Annals of Internal Medicine* 142 (2005): 37–46.

21. "Segment Profile: Vitamins & Minerals," 1–4.

22. Kathy Radimer, Bernadette Bindewald, Jeffrey Hughes, Bethene Ervin, Christine Swanson, and Mary Frances Picciano, "Dietary Supplement Use by US Adults: Data from the National Health and Nutrition Examination Survey, 1999–2000," *American Journal of Epidemiology* 160 (2004): 339–349.

23. Cuiwei Zhao, Karen W. Andrews, Joanne M. Holden, Amy L. Schweitzer, Janet Roseland, James Harnly, Wayne Wolf, Johanna T. Dwyer, Mary Frances Picciano, Joseph M. Betz, Leila G. Saldanha, Elizabeth Yetley, Kenneth Fisher, Kathy Radimer, "Antioxidant Supplements Reported in the National Health and Nutrition Examination Survey (NHANES)," U.S. Department of Agriculture, 1999–2000, http://www.nal.usda.gov/fnic/foodcomp/Data/Other/AICR05_AntioxidantSupp.pdf (accessed May 16, 2007).

24. Radimer et al., "Dietary Supplement Use by US Adults": 339–349; Millen, et al., "Use of Vitamin, Mineral, Nonvitamin, and Nonmineral Supplements in the United

States": 942–950; American Dietetic Association, "Nutrition and You: Trends 2000": 626–627.

25. Babgaleh B. Timbo, Marianne P. Ross, Patrick V. McCarthy, and Chung-Tung J. Ling, "Dietary Supplements in a National Survey: Prevalence of Use and Reports of Adverse Events," *Journal of the American Dietetic Association* 106, no. 12 (December 2006): 1966–1974.

26. Food and Nutrition Board, *Dietary Supplements: A Framework for Evaluating Safety.*

27. Ibid.

28. Vicki Brower, "A Nutraceutical a Day May Keep the Doctor Away," *EMBRO Reports* 6, no. 8 (2005): 708–711, http://www.pubmedcentral.nih.gov/articlerender.fcgi?tool=pmcentrez&artid=1369156 (accessed January 10, 2007).

29. Vicky Newman, Cheryl L. Rock, Susan Faerber, Shirley W. Flatt, Fred A. Wright, and John P. Pierce, "Dietary Supplement Use by Women at Risk for Breast Cancer Recurrence," *Journal of the American Dietetic Association* 98, no. 3 (March 1998): 285–292, http://www.adajournal.org/article/PIIS0002822398000686/fulltext (accessed January 10, 2007); A. J. Satia-About, A. R. Kristal, R. E. Patterson, A. J. Littman, K. L. Stratton, and E. White, "Dietary Supplement Use and Medical Conditions: The VITAL Study," *American Journal of Preventive Medicine* 24 (2003): 43–51: http://download.journals.elsevierhealth.com/pdfs/journals/0749-3797/O11S0749379702005718.pdf (accessed March 4, 2007).

30. Food and Nutrition Board, *"Dietary Supplements: A Framework for Evaluating Safety."*

31. Erica Frank, "Physician Health and Patient Care," *Journal of American Medical Association* 291 (2004): 637, http://jama.ama-assn.org/cgi/content/full/291/5/637 (accessed January 14, 2007).

32. Vincent Wahner-Roedler, Peter L. Elkin, Laura L. Loehrer, Stephen S. Cha, and Brent A. Bauer, "Physicians' Attitudes toward Complementary and Alternative Medicine and Their Knowledge of Specific Therapies: A Survey at an Academic Medical Center," *Oxford Journal* 3, no. 4 (2006): 495–501, http://ecam.oxfordjournals.org/cgi/content/full/3/4/495 (accessed January 14, 2007).

33. E. Frank, A. Bendich, and M. Denniston, "Use of Vitamin-Mineral Supplements by Female Physicians in the United States," *American Journal of Clinical Nutrition* 72, no. 4 (October 2000): 969–975, http://www.ajcn.org/cgi/content/full/72/4/969?ck=nck (accessed May 16, 1997).

34. Timbo et al., "Dietary Supplements in a National Survey, 1966–1974."

35. Ibid.

36. W. C. Willett and M. J. Stampfer, "Clinical Practice: What Vitamins Should I Be Taking, Doctor?" *NE J Med* 345 (2001): 1819–1824; R. H. Fletcher and K. M. Fairfield, "Vitamins for Chronic Disease Prevention in Adults: Scientific Review," *Journal of American Medical Association* 287 (2002): 3116–3126.

37. Food and Nutrition Board, Institute of Medicine of the National Academies, *Dietary Reference Intakes for Vitamin C, Vitamin E, Selenium, and Carotenoids.* Washington, DC: National Academy Press, 2000.

38. G. S. Omenn, G. E. Goodman, M. D. Thornquist, J. Balmes, M. R. Cullen, A. Glass, J. P. Keogh, F. L. Meyskens, Jr., B. Valanis, J. H. Williams, Jr., S. Barnhart, M. G. Cherniack, C. A. Brodkin, and S. Hammar, "Risk Factors Lung Cancer and for

Intervention Effects in CARET, the Beta-Carotene and Retinol Efficacy Trial," *Journal of the National Cancer Institute* 88, no. 21 (November 6, 1996): 1550–1559.

39. National Institutes of Health, "NIH State-of-the-Science Conference Statement."

40. Ibid.

CHAPTER 2

1. Elmer Verner McCollum, *A History of Nutrition*, Boston: Houghton Mifflin Co., 1957, 3.

2. George Wolf, "A Historical Note on the Mode of Administration of Vitamin A for the Cure of Night Blindness," *American Journal of Clinical Nutrition* 31 (February 1978): 290–292, http://www.ajcn.org/cgi/reprint/31/2/290.pdf (accessed March 22, 2007).

3. McCollum, *A History of Nutrition*, 266–267.

4. Ibid., 1–7.

5. Daniel NIV. The Book of Daniel 1:18, *The NIV Study Bible*, 10th Anniversary Edition, Grand Rapids, MI: Zondervan Publishing House, 1995, 1291.

6. Helen Andrews Guthrie, "Overview of Nutrition," *Introductory Nutrition*, St. Louis: The C.V. Mosby Co., 1975, 4.

7. Harvard School of Public Health, "Vitamins," *Harvard College*, 2007, http://www.hsph.harvard.edu/nutritionsource/vitamins.html (accessed March 7, 2007).

8. Marcel Trudel, "Cartier, Jacques," Dictionary of Canadian Biography Online, Library and Archives Canada, University of Toronto, 2000, http://www.biographi.ca/EN/ShowBio.asp?Biold=34229 (accessed May 27, 2007).

9. Guthrie, *Introductory Nutrition*, 237; "History Highlights of Nutrition," http://www.ansc.purdue.edu/courses/ansc221v/histnote.htm (accessed March 22, 2007).

10. "History Highlights of Nutrition;" McCollum, *A History of Nutrition*, 215–216.

11. Guthrie, *Introductory Nutrition*, 4–5.

12. Center for Human Nutrition, "History," *John Hopkins Bloomberg School of Public Health*, 2005, http://www.jhsph.edu/chn/About%20US/history.html (accessed January 22, 2007); Guthrie, *Introductory Nutrition*, 4–5.

13. Guthrie, *Introductory Nutrition*, 4–5.

14. Ibid., 10.

15. Ibid., 197.

16. Ibid., 197–201.

17. Carl E. Anderson, "Minerals," *Nutritional Support of Medical Practice*. Maryland: Harper & Row, 1977, 57–72.

18. Food and Nutrition Board, Institute of Medicine of the National Academies, *Dietary Reference Intakes for Vitamin C, Vitamin E, Selenium, and Carotenoids*, Washington, DC: National Academy Press, 2000, 17.

19. R. E. Hughes, "Nonfoods as Dietary Supplements," *The Cambridge World History of Food*, Cambridge University Press, 2000, http://www.cambridge.org/us/books/kiple/nonfoods.htm (accessed March 22, 2007).

20. Jennifer J. Otten, Jennifer P. Hellwig, and Linda D. Meyers, "Introduction to the Dietary Reference Intakes," *Dietary Reference Intakes: The Essential Guide to Nutrient Requirements*, Washington, DC: The National Academies Press, 2006, 5–6.

21. Ibid.

22. Ibid., 6–68.

23. Wallace F. Janssen, "The Story of the Laws behind the Labels, Part I," *FDA Consumer*, June 1981, http://www.cfsan.fda.gov/~lrd/history1.html (accessed January 30, 2007).

24. Wallace F. Janssen, "The Story of the Laws behind the Labels, Part II," *FDA Consumer*, June 1981, http://www.cfsan.fda.gov/~lrd/history1.html (accessed January 30, 2007).

25. CFSAN/Office of Food Additive Safety, "Guidance for Industry Frequently Asked Questions About GRAS," U.S. Food and Drug Administration, College Park, Maryland, December 2004, http://www.cfsan.fda.gov/~dms/grasguid.html#Q (accessed May 17, 2007).

26. Wallace F. Janssen, "The Story of the Laws behind the Labels, Part III," *FDA Consumer*, June 1981, http://www.cfsan.fda.gov/~lrd/history1.html (accessed January 30, 2007); Janssen, *FDA Consumer*, Part I.

27. Center for Food Safety and Applied Nutrition, " Dietary Supplement Health and Education Act of 1994," U.S. Food and Drug Administration, College Park, Maryland, December 1, 1995, http://www.cfsan.fda.gov/~dms/dietsupp.html (accessed March 11, 2007).

28. Ibid.

29. Ibid.

30. Office of Dietary Supplements, "About the Office of Dietary Supplements (ODS)," National Institutes of Health (NIH), Bethesda, MD, http://ods.od.nih.gov/about/about_ods.aspx (accessed May 7, 2007).

31. NIH, "The NIH Almanac–Organization," U.S. Department of Health and Human Services, 2007, http://www.nih.gov/about/almanac/organization/NCCAM.htm (accessed May 7, 2007).

32. June Weintraub, "Adverse Effects of Botanical and Non-Botanical Ephedrine Products," *Harvard School of Public Health*, 1997, http://www.hsph.harvard.edu/Organizations/DDIL/ephedrine.html (accessed March 11, 2007); U.S. Food and Drug Administration, "FDA Issues Regulation Prohibiting Sale of Dietary Supplements Containing Ephedrine Alkaloids and Reiterates Its Advice That Consumers Stop Using These Products," *FDA News*, February 6, 2004, http://www.cfsan.fda.gov/~lrd/fpephed6.html (accessed March 11, 2007); "Ephedra Side Effects," Ephedrine News, http://www.ephedrine-news.com/html/effects.html (accessed May 19, 2007); Sidney M. Wolfe, "Statement on HHS Failure to Ban Ephedra or Issue Adequate Warnings (HRG Publication #1624)," Public Citizen, June 14, 2000, http://www.citizen.org/publications/release.cfm?ID=7180 (accessed May 19, 2007); "Questions and Answers about FDA's Actions on Dietary Supplements Containing Ephedrine Alkaloids," U.S. Food and Drug Administration, February 6, 2004, http://www.fda.gov/oc/initiatives/ephera/february2004/qa_020604.html (accessed May 19, 2007); "Ephedra Side Effects News," Ephedrine News, http://www.ephedrine-news.com (accessed May 19, 2007); Marcia Crosse, "Dietary Supplements Containing Ephedra. Health Risks and FDA's Oversight," General Accounting Office, July 23, 2003, http://www.gao.gov/new.items/d031042t.pdf (accessed May 19, 2007).

33. "Consumers Warned of Problems with Multivitamins," ConsumerLab.com, January 19, 2007, http://www.consumerlab.com/news/news_011907_multivitamin.asp (accessed May 19, 2007).

CHAPTER 3

1. Z. Seward, "Quest for Youth Drives Craze for 'Wine' Pills," *The Wall Street Journal,* November 30, 2006.
2. K. T. Howitz, K. J. Bitterman, H. Y. Cohen, D. W. Lamming, S. Lavu, J. G. Wood, R. E. Zipkin, P. Chung, A. Kisielewski, L-L. Zhang, B. Scherer, and D. A. Sinclair, "Small Molecule Activators of Sirtuins Extend Saccharomyces Cerevisiae Lifespan," *Nature* 425 (2003): 191–196.
3. J. A. Baur, K. J. Pearson, N. L. Price, H. A. Jamieson, C. Lerin, A. Kalra, V. V. Prabhu, J. S. Allard, G. Lopez-Lluch, K. Lewis, P. J. Pistell, S. Poosala, K. G. Becker, O. Boss, D. Gwinn, M. Wang, S. Ramaswamy, K. W. Fishbein, R. G. Spencer, E. G. Lakatta, D. Le Couteur, R. J. Shaw, P. Navas, P. Puigserver, D. K. Ingram, R.l de Cabo, and D. A. Sinclair, "Resveratrol Improves Health and Survival of Mice on a High-Calorie Diet," *Nature* 444 (2006): 337–342.
4. B. Halliwell and J. M. C. Gutteridge, *Free Radicals in Biology and Medicine*, 4th ed., Oxford: Clarendon Press, 2006.
5. M. Gomberg, "An Instance of Trivalent Carbon: Triphenylmethyl," *Journal of American Chemical Society* 22, no. 11 (1900): 757–771.
6. D. Harman, "Ageing: A Theory based on Free Radical and Radiation Chemistry," *Journal of Gerontology* 2 (1957): 298–300.
7. W. A. Pryor, "Organic Free Radicals," *Chemical Engineering News* 24 (1968): 70–89.
8. J. M. McCord and Fridovich, "The Reduction of Cytochrome C by Milk Xanthine Oxidase," *Journal of Biological Chemistry* 243 (1968): 5753–5760.
9. R. M. Lebovitz, H. Zhang, H. Vogel, Dionne L. Cartwright, Jr, N. Lu, S. Huang, and M. M Matzuk, "Neurodegeneration, Myocardial Injury, and Perinatal Death in Mitochondrial Superoxide Dismutase-deficient Mice," *Proceedings of the National Academy of Sciences of the USA* 93 (1996): 9782–9787.
10. International Union of Pure and Applied Chemistry, Organic Chemistry Division, "Sections A, B, C, D, E, F and H," *Commission on Nomenclature of Organic Chemistry, Nomenclature of Organic Chemistry,* Oxford: Pergamon Press, 1979, 559.
11. W. H. Koppenol, "What Is in a Name? Rules for Radicals," *Free Radical Biology and Medicine* 9 (1990): 225–227.
12. W. H. Koppenol, "Names for Inorganic Radicals," *Pure and Applied Chemistry* 72 (2000): 437–446; J. G. Traynham, "A Short Guide to Nomenclature of Radicals, Radical Ions, Iron-oxygen Complexes and Polycyclic Aromatic Hydrocarbons," *Advanced Free Radical Biology and Medicine* 2 (1986): 191–209; Koppenol, "NO Nomenclature," *Nitric Oxide Biological Chemistry* 6 (2002): 96–98.
13. T. M. Millar, "Peroxynitrite Formation from the Simultaneous Reduction of Nitrite and Oxygen by Xanthine Oxidase," *FEBS Letters* 562, no. 1–3 (March 26, 2004): 129–133.
14. Food and Nutrition Board, Institute of Medicine of the National Academies, *Dietary Reference Intakes for Vitamin C, Vitamin E, Selenium, and Carotenoids.* Washington, DC: National Academy Press, 2000.
15. B. Halliwell and J. M. C. Gutteridge, "The Definition and Measurement of Antioxidants in Biological Systems," *Free Radical Biology and Medicine* 18 (1995): 125–126.
16. G. R. Buettner, "The Pecking Order of Free Radicals and Antioxidants: Lipid Peroxidation, a-tocopherol, and Ascorbate," *Archives of Biochemistry and Biophysics* 2 (1993): 535–543.

17. N. Smirnoff, P. L Conklin, and F. A. Loewus, "Biosynthesis of Ascorbic Acid in Plants: A Renaissance," *Annual Review of Plant Physiology and Plant Molecular Biology* 52 (June 2001): 437–467.

18. Ibid.

19. N. Tanuguchi, T. Higashi, Y. Sakamoto, A. Meister (eds.), *Glutathione Centennial: Molecular Perspectives and Clinical Implications.* New York: Academic Press, 1989.

20. A. Meister, "On the Antioxidant Effect of Ascorbic Acid and Glutathione," *Biochem Pharmacology* 44 (1992): 1905–1915.

21. M. R. McCall and B. Frei, "Can Antioxidant Vitamins Materially Reduce Oxidative Damage in Humans?" *Free Radical Biology and Medicine* 26 (1999): 1034–1053; S. Loft and H.E. Poulsen, "Antioxidant Intervention Studies Related to DNA Damage, DNA Repair and Gene Expression," *Free Radical Research* 33 (2000): S67–S83; L. J. Roberts, 2nd, and J. D. Morrow, "Products of the Isoprostane Pathway: Unique Bioactive Compounds and Markers of Lipid Peroxidation," *Cellular and Molecular Life Sciences* 59 (2002): 808–820.

22. V. W. Bowry and R. Stocker, "Tocopherol-mediated Peroxidation. The Prooxidant Effect of Vitamin E on the Radical-initiated Oxidation of Human Low-density Lipoprotein," *Journal of American Chemical Society* 115 (1993): 6029–6040.

23. Halliwell and Gutteridge, *Free Radicals in Biology and Medicine.*

24. B. Halliwell, "Free Radicals, Antioxidants, and Human Disease: Curiosity, Cause, or Consequence?" *Lancet* 344 (September 10, 1994): 721–724.

25. A. H. Knoll and H. D. Holland, "Oxygen and Proterozoic Evolution: An Update," *Panel on Effects of Past Global Change on Life, National Research Council. Effects of Past Global Change on Life.* Washington, DC: National Academies Press, 1995, 272.

26. J. Raymond and D. Segre, "The Effect of Oxygen on Biochemical Networks and the Evolution of Complex Life," *Science* 24, no. 311 (March 2006): 1764–1767.

27. J. M. Hayes, "A Lowdown on Oxygen," *Nature* 417 (2002): 127–128.

28. J. F. Kasting, "Earth's Early Atmosphere," *Science* 259 (1993): 920–926.

29. B. Wiedenheft, J. Mosolf, D. Willits, M. Yeager, K.A. Dryden, M. Young, and T. Douglas, "An Archaeal Antioxidant: Characterization of a Dps-like Protein from Sulfolobus solfataricus," *Proceedings of the National Academy of Sciences of the USA* 102 (2005): 10551–10556.

30. C. P. Mangum, "Major Events in the Evolution of the Oxygen Carriers," *American Zoology* 38 (1998):1–13.

31. D. C. Chow, L. A.Wenning, W. M. Miller, and E. T. Papoutsakis, "Modeling pO(2) Distributions in the Bone Marrow Hematopoietic Compartment. I. Krogh's Model," *Biophysical Journal* 81 (2001): 675–684.

32. G. Barja, "Mitochondrial Oxygen Radical Generation and Leak: Sites of Production in States 4 and 3, Organ Specificity, and Relation to Aging and Longevity," *Journal of Bioenergetics Biomembranes* 31, no. 4 (August 31, 1999): 347–366.

33. R. B. Johnston, Jr., and S. Kitagawa, "Molecular Basis for the Enhanced Respiratory Burst of Activated Macrophages," *Federation Proceedings* 44, no. 14 (1985): 2927–2932.

34. B. Halliwell, "Reactive Species and Antioxidants. Redox Biology is a Fundamental Theme of Aerobic Life," *Plant Physiology* 141, no. 2 (June 2006): 312–322.

35. R. E. Blankenship and H. Hartman, "The Origin and Evolution of Oxygenic Photosynthesis," *Trends in Biochemical Sciences* 23 (1998): 94–97.

36. Halliwell, "Reactive Species and Antioxidants."

37. M. G. Klotz and P. C. Loewen, "The Molecular Evolution of Catalatic Hydroperoxidases: Evidence for Multiple Lateral Transfer of Genes between Prokaryota and from Bacteria into Eukaryota," *Molecular Biology and Evolution* 20, no. 7 (2003): 1098–1112.

38. J. M. Olson and R.E. Blankenship, "Thinking about the Evolution of Photosynthesis," *Photosynthesis Research* 80 (2004): 373–386.

39. R. A. Berner and D. E. Canfield, "A New Model for Atmospheric Oxygen over Phanerozoic Time," *American Journal of Science* 289 (1989): 333–361.

40. J. Graham, R. Dudley, N. Aguilar, and C. Gans, "Implications of the Late Palaeozoic Oxygen Pulse for Physiology and Evolution," *Nature* 375 (1995): 117–120.

41. K. Malkowski, M. Gruszczynski, A. Hoffman, and S. Halas, "Oceanic Stable Isotope Composition and a Scenario for the Permo-Triassic Crisis," *Historical Biology* 2 (1989): 289–309.

42. D. J. Beerling, F. I. Woodward, M. R.Lomas, M. A. Wills, W. P. Quick, and P. J. Valdes, "The Influence of Carboniferous Palaeoatmospheres on Plant Function: An Experimental and Modelling Assessment," *Philosophical Transactions of the Royal Society. Series B: Biological Sciences* 353 (1998): 131–139.

43. I. Fridovich, "Superoxide Radical and SODs," *Annual Review of Biochemistry* 64 (1995): 97–112.

44. A. W. Girotti, "Photosensitized Oxidation of Cholesterol in Biological-systems—Reaction Pathways, Cytotoxic Effects and Defense Mechanisms," *Journal of Photochemistry and Photobiology. B Biology* 13 (1992): 105–118; G. D. Ouedraogo and R. W. Redmond, "Secondary Reactive Oxygen Species Extend the Range of Photosensitization Effects in Cells: DNA Damage Produced via Initial Membrane Photosensitization," *Photochemistry and Photobiology* 77 (2003): 192–203.

45. N. E. Holt, D. Zigmantas, L.Valkunas, X. P. Li, K. K. Niyogi, and G. R. Fleming, "Carotenoid Cation Formation and the Regulation of Photosynthetic Light Harvesting," *Science* 307 (2005): 433–436.

46. M. Szibor and J. Holtz, "Mitochondrial Ageing," *Basic Research in Cardiology* 98, no. 4 (July 2003): 210–218; G. T. Babcock, "How Oxygen is Activated and Reduced in Respiration," *Proceedings of the National Academy of Sciences of the USA* 96 (1999): 13114–13117.

47. M. D. Brand, C. Affourtit, T. C. Esteves, K. Green, A. J. Lambert, S. Miwa, J. L. Pakay, and N. Parker, "Mitochondrial Superoxide: Production, Biological Effects, and Activation of Uncoupling Proteins," *Free Radical Biology and Medicine* 37 (2004): 755–767.

48. Fridovich, "Superoxide Radical and SODs."

49. R. Brigelius-Flohe, "Tissue-specific Functions of Individual Glutathione Peroxidases," *Free Radical Biology and Medicine* 27 (1999): 951–965.

50. S. G. Rhee, H. Z. Chae, and K. Kim, "Peroxiredoxins: A Historical Overview and Speculative Preview of Novel Mechanisms and Emerging Concepts in Cell Signaling," *Free Radical Biology and Medicine* 38: 1543–1552.

51. G. F. Combs, Jr., and S. B. Combs, "The Nutritional Biochemistry of Selenium," *Annual Review of Nutrition* 4 (2005): 257–280.

52. M. G. Traber and L. Packer, "Vitamin E: Beyond Antioxidant Function," *American Journal of Clinical Nutrition* 62, no. 6 supp (December 1995): 1501S–1509S.

53. S. Ohno, "Evolution by Gene Duplication," *Springer-Verlag*, New York, 1970; T. Blomme, K. Vandepoele, S. De Bodt, C. Simillion, S. Maere, and Y. Van de Peer, "The

Gain and Loss of Genes during 600 Million Years of Vertebrate Evolution," *Genome Biology* 7, no. 5 (2006): R43.

54. M Nishikimi, R. Fukuyama, S. Minoshima, N. Shimizu, and K. Yagi, "Cloning and Chromosomal Mapping of the Human Nonfunctional Gene for L-gulono-gamma-lactone Oxidase, the Enzyme for L-ascorbic Acid Biosynthesis Missing in Man," *Journal of Biological Chemistry* 269, no. 18 (1994): 13685–13688.

55. R. A. Weale, "Biorepair Mechanisms and Longevity," *Journal of Gerontology Series A: Biological Sciences and Medical Sciences* 59 (May 2004): B449–B454.

CHAPTER 4

1. W. A. Pryor, "Vitamin E and Heart Disease: Basic Science to Clinical Intervention Trials," *Free Radical Biology & Medicine* 28, no. 1 (January 1, 2000): 141–164.

2. A. P. Pillay, "Vitamin-C Test for Ovulation," *Human Fertility* 2, no. 4 (1946): 109–110.

3. C. Funk, "Studies on Beri-beri: VII. Chemistry of the Vitamine-fraction from Yeast and Rice-polishings," *Journal of Physiology* 46, no. 3 (June 19, 1913): 173–179.

4. A. Szent-Györgyi, "On the Mechanism of Biological Oxidation and the Function of the Suprarenal," *Science* (August 1, 1930): 125–126.

5. C. G. King and W. A. Waugh, "The Chemical Nature of Vitamin C," *Science* 75 (April 1932): 357–358; Otto A. Bessey and C. G. King, "The Distribution of Vitamin C in Plant and Animal Tissues, and its Determination," *Journal of Biological Chemistry* 103 (December 1933): 687–698.

6. E. S. McCluskey, "Which Vertebrates Make Vitamin C?" *Origins* 12, no. 2 (1985): 96–100.

7. D. J. Prockop and K.I. Kivirikko, "Collagens: Molecular Biology, Diseases, and Potentials for Therapy," *Annual Review of Biochemistry* 64 (1995): 403–434.

8. C. J. Rebouche, "Ascorbic Acid and Carnitine Biosynthesis," *American Journal of Clinical Nutrition* 54, no. 6 suppl (1991): 1147S–1152S.

9. Levine M. Hartzell and A. Bdolah, "Ascorbic Acid and Mg-ATP Co-regulate Dopamine Beta-monooxygenase Activity in Intact Chromaffin Granules," *Journal of Biological Chemistry* 263, no. 263 (1988): 19353–19362.

10. Y. I. Miller, M. K. Chang, C. J. Binder, P. X. Shaw, and J. L. Witztum, "Oxidized Low Density Lipoprotein and Innate Immune Receptors," *Current Opinion in Lipidology* 14, no. 5 (October 2003): 437–445; J. Fan and T. Watanabe, "Inflammatory Reactions in the Pathogenesis of Atherosclerosis," *Journal of Atherosclerosis and Thrombosis* 10, no. 2 (2003): 63–71.

11. M. N. Diaz, B. Frei, J. A. Vita, J. F. Keaney. "Antioxidants and Atherosclerotic Heart Disease," *New England Journal of Medicine* 337 (1997): 408–416; I. Jialal and C. J. Fuller, "Oxidatively Modified LDL and Atherosclerosis: An Evolving Plausible Scenario," *Critical Reviews in Food Science and Nutrition* 36, no. 4 (April 1996): 341–355; N. K. Andrikopoulos, A. C. Kaliora, A. N. Assimopoulou, and V. P. Papageorgiou, "Inhibitory Activity of Minor Polyphenolic and Non-polyphenolic Constituents of Olive Oil against In vitro Low-density Lipoprotein Oxidation," *Journal of Medicinal Food* 5 (2002): 1–7.

12. P. Milbury, C. Y. Chen, J. K. Kwak, and J. Blumberg, "Almond Skins Polyphenolics Act Synergistically with alpha-Tocopherol to Increase the Resistance of Low-density Lipoproteins to Oxidation," *Free Radical Research* 36, Supp/1 (2002): 78–79.

13. F. B. Hu, "The Iron-heart Hypothesis: Search for the Ironclad Evidence," *JAMA* 297, no. 6 (February 14, 2007): 639–641.

14. J. L. Sullivan, "Iron and the Sex Difference in Heart Disease Risk," *Lancet* 1 (1981): 1293–1294.

15. M. A. Livrea, L. Tesoriere, A. M. Pintaudi, A. Calabrese, A. Maggio, H. J. Freisleben, D. D'Arpa, R. D'Anna, and A. Bongiorno, "Oxidative Stress and Antioxidant Status in beta-Thalassemia Major: Iron Overload and Depletion of Lipid-soluble Antioxidants," *Blood* 88, no. 9 (November 1, 1996): 3608–36014.

16. M. R. McCall and B. Frei, "Can Antioxidant Vitamins Materially Reduce Oxidative Damage in Humans?" *Free Radical Biology & Medicine* 7–8 (April 26, 1999): 1034–1053.

17. M. J. Stampfer, C. H. Hennekens, J. E. Manson, G. A. Colditz, B. Rosner, W. C. Willett, "Vitamin E Consumption and the Risk of Coronary Disease in Women," *New England Journal of Medicine* 328 (1993):1444–1449.

18. E. B. Rimm, M. J. Stampfer, A. Ascherio, E. Giovannucci, G. A. Colditz, and W. C. Willett, "Vitamin E Consumption and the Risk of Coronary Heart Disease in Men," *New England Journal of Medicine* 328 (1993): 1450–1456.

19. J. E. Enstrom, L. E. Kanim, and M. A. Klein, "Vitamin C Intake and Mortality among a Sample of the United States Population," *Epidemiology* 3 (1992): 194–202.

20. "The Effect of Vitamin E and Beta Carotene on the Incidence of Lung Cancer and Other Cancers in Male Smokers. The Alpha-Tocopherol, Beta Carotene Cancer Prevention Study Group," *New England Journal of Medicine* 330, no. 15 (April 14, 1994): 1029–1035.

21. J. M. Leppala, J. Virtamo, R. Fogelholm, J. K. Huttunen, D. Albanes, P. R. Taylor, and O. P. Heinonen, "Controlled Trial of Alpha-tocopherol and Beta-carotene Supplements on Stroke Incidence and Mortality in Male Smokers." *Arteriosclerosis, Thrombosis, and Vascular Biology* 20, no. 1 (January 2000): 230–235.

22. G. S. Omenn, G. E. Goodman, M. D. Thornquist, J. Balmes, M. R. Cullen, A. Glass, J. P. Keogh, F. L. Meyskens, B. Valanis, J. H. Williams, S. Barnhart, and S. Hammar, "Effects of a Combination of Beta Carotene and Vitamin A on Lung Cancer and Cardiovascular Disease," *New England Journal of Medicine* 334, no. 18 (May 1996): 1150–1155.

23. C. H. Hennekens, J. E. Buring, J. E. Manson, M. Stampfer, B. Rosner, N.R. Cook, C. Belanger, F. LaMotte, J. M. Gaziano, P. M. Ridker, W. Willett, and R. Peto, "Lack of Effect of Long-term Supplementation with Beta Carotene on the Incidence of Malignant Neoplasms and Cardiovascular Disease," *New England Journal of Medicine* 334 (1996): 1145–1149.

24. M. Levine, "New Concepts in the Biology and Biochemistry of Ascorbic Acid," *New England Journal of Medicine* 314 (1986): 892–902.

25. K. F. Gey, G. B. Brubacher, and H. B. Stahelin, "Plasma Levels of Antioxidant Vitamins in Relation to Ischemic Heart Disease and Cancer," *American Journal of Clinical Nutrition* 45 (1987): 1368.

26. A. C. Carr and B. Frei, "Toward a New Recommended Dietary Allowance for Vitamin C based on Antioxidant and Health Effects in Humans," *American Journal of Clinical Nutrition* 69, no. 6 (1999): 1086–1107.

27. M. Levine, K. R. Dhariwal, R. W. Welch, Y. Wang, and J. B. Park, "Determination of Optimal Vitamin C Requirements in Humans," *American Journal of Clinical Nutrition* 62 (December 1995): 1347–1356.

28. G. Schectman, J. C Byrd, and R. Hoffmann, "Ascorbic Acid Requirements for Smokers: Analysis of a Population Survey," *American Journal of Clinical Nutrition* 53, no. 6 (1991): 1466–1470.

29. J. Zhang, X. Ying, Q. Lu, A. Kallner, R.-J. Xiu, P. Henriksson, and I. Björkhem, "A Single High Dose of Vitamin C Counteracts the Acute Negative Effect on Microcirculation Induced by Smoking a Cigarette," *Microvascular Research* 58, no. 3 (November 1999): 305–311.

30. C. S. Johnston, "Biomarkers for Establishing a Tolerable Upper Intake Level for Vitamin C," *Nutrition Reviews* 57, no. 3 (March 1999): 71–77.

31. A. Bendich and L. Langseth, "The Health Effects of Vitamin C Supplementation: A Review," *Journal of American College of Nutrition* 14, no. 2 (April 1995): 124–136.

32. J. E. Enstrom, L. E. Kanim, and M. A. Klein, "Vitamin C Intake and Mortality among a Sample of the United States Population," *Epidemiology* 3, no. 3 (1992): 194–202; C. Fortes, F. Forastiere, S. Farchi, E. Rapiti, G. Pastori, and C. A. Perucci, "Diet and Overall Survival in a Cohort of Very Elderly People," *Epidemiology* 11, no. 4 (July 2000): 440–445; P. Mecocci, M. C. Polidori, L. Troiano, A. Cherubini, R. Cecchetti, G. Pini, M. Straatman, D. Monti, W. Stahl, H. Sies, C. Franceschi, and U. Senin, "Plasma Antioxidants and Longevity: A Study on Healthy Centenarians," *Free Radical Biology & Medicine* 25, no. 8 (April 15, 2000): 1243–1248.

33. P. F. Jacques, A. Taylor, S. E. Hankinson, W. C. Willett, B. Mahnken, Y. Lee, K. Vaid, and M. Lahav, "Long-term Vitamin C Supplement Use and Prevalence of Early Age-related Lens Opacities," *American Journal of Clinical Nutrition* 66, no. 4 (October 1997): 911–916.

34. A. Taylor, P. F. Jacques, D. Nadler, F. Morrow, S. I. Sulsky, and D. Shepard, "Relationship in Humans between Ascorbic Acid Consumption and Levels of Total and Reduced Ascorbic Acid in Lens, Aqueous Humor, and Plasma," *Current Eye Research* 10, no. 8 (August 1991): 751–759.

35. R. E. Koes, F. Quattrocchio, and N. M. Joseph, "The Flavonoid Biosynthetic Pathway in Plants: Function and Evolution," *Molecular Biology Essays* 16 (1994): 123–132.

36. D. A. Smith and S. W. Banks, "Biosynthesis, Elicitation and Biological Activity of Isoflavonoid Phytoalexins," *Phytochemistry* 25 (1986): 979–995.

37. S. A. J. Zaat, C. A. Wijffelman, H. P. Spaink, A. A. van Brussel, R. J. Okker, and B. J. Lugtenberg, "Induction of the NodA Promoter of Rhizobium Leguminosarum Symplasmid pRLIJI by Plant Flavanones and Flavones," *Journal of Bacteriology* 169 (1987): 198–204.

38. K. R. Price, J. R. Bacon, and M. J. C. Rhodes, "Effect of Storage and Domestic Processing on the Content and Composition of Flavonol Glucosides in Onion (Allium cepa)," *Journal of Agricultural and Food Chemistry* 15 (1997): 938–942.

39. G. Williamson and C. Manach, "Bioavailability and Bioefficacy of Polyphenols in Humans. II. Review of 93 Intervention Studies," *American Journal of Clinical Nutrition* 81 (2005): 243S–255S.

40. C. Manach, A. Scalbert, C. Morand, C. Remesy, and L. Jimenez, "Polyphenols: Food Sources and Bioavailability," *American Journal of Clinical Nutrition* 79 (2004): 727–747.

41. W. Bors, C. Michel, and K. Stettmaier, "Structure-activity Relationships Governing Antioxidant Capacities of Plant Polyphenols," *Methods in Enzymology* 335 (2001): 166–180.

42. I. M. Zijp, O. Korver, and L. B. M. Tijburg, "Effect of Tea and Other Dietary Factors on Iron Absorption," *Critical Reviews in Food Science and Nutrition* 40 (2000): 371–398.

43. M. E. Widlansky, S. J. Duffy, N. M. Hamburg, N. Gokce, B. A. Warden, S. Wiseman, J. F. Keaney, B. Frei, and J. A. Vita, "Effects of Black Tea Consumption on Plasma Catechins and Markers of Oxidative Stress and Inflammation in Patients with Coronary Artery Disease," *Free Radical Biology & Medicine* 38 (2005): 499–506; I. Wiswedel, D. Hirsch, S. Kropf, M. Gruening, E. Pfister, T. Schewe, and H. Sies, "Flavanol-rich Cocoa Drink Lowers Plasma F2-Isoprostane Concentrations in Humans," *Free Radical Biology & Medicine* 37 (2004): 411–421; M. E. Lean, M. Noroozi, I. Kelly, J. Burns, D. Talwar, N. Sattar, and A. Crozier, "Dietary Flavonols Protect Diabetic Human Lymphocytes against Oxidative Damage to DNA," *Diabetes* 48 (1999): 176–181.

44. P. Milbury, C-Y. Chen, H-K. Kwak, and J. Blumberg, "Almond Skins Polyphenolics Act Synergistically with α-Tocopherol to Increase the Resistance of Low-density Lipoproteins to Oxidation," *Free Radical Research* 36, S (2002): 78–80.

45. A. N. Kong, E. Owuor, R. Yu, V. Hebbar, C. Chen, R. Hu, and S. Mandlekar, "Induction of Xenobiotic Enzymes by the MAP Kinase Pathway and the Antioxidant or Electrophile Response Element (ARE/EpRE)," *Drug Metabolism Reviews* 33 (2001): 255–271.

46. P. E. Milbury, B. Graf, J. M. Curran-Celentano, and J. B. Blumberg, "Bilberry (Vaccinium myrtillus) Anthocyanins Modulate Heme Oxygenase-1 and Glutathione S-Transferase-pi Expression in ARPE-19 Cells," *Investigative Ophthalmology and Visual Science* 48, no. 5 (May 2007): 2343–2349.

47. Y. Zhang and G. M. Gordon, "A Strategy for Cancer Prevention: Stimulation of the Nrf2-ARE Signaling Pathway," *Molecular Cancer Therapy* 3 (2004): 885–893.

48. R. J. Williams, J. P. E. Spencer, and C. Rice-Evans, "Flavonoids: Antioxidants or Signaling Molecules?" *Free Radical Biology & Medicine* 36 (2004): 838–849.

49. E. Middleton Jr., C. Kandaswami, and T. C. Theoharides, "The Effects of Plant Flavonoids on Mammalian Cells: Implications for Inflammation, Heart Disease, and Cancer," *Pharmacological Reviews* 52 (2000): 673–751.

50. F. Hollosyand and G. Keri, "Plant-derived Protein Tyrosine Kinase Inhibitors as Anticancer Agents," *Current Medicinal Chemistry of Anti-Cancer Agents* 4 (2004): 173–197.

51. M. G. Hertog, D. Kromhout, C. Aravanis, H. Blackburn, R. Buzina, F. Fidanza, S. Giampaoli, A. Jansen, A. Menotti, S. Nedeljkovic, M. Pekkarinen, B. S. Simic, H. Toshima, E. J. Feskens, P. C. Hollman, and M. B. Katan, "Flavonoid Intake and Long-term Risk of Coronary Heart Disease and Cancer in the Seven Countries Study," *Archives of Internal Medicine* 155 (1995): 381–386.

52. K. Maeda, M. Kuzuya, X. W. Cheng, T. Asai, S. Kanda, N. Tamaya-Mori, T. Sasaki, T. Shibata, and A. Iguchi, "Green Tea Catechins Inhibit the Cultured Smooth Muscle Cell Invasion through the Basement Barrier," *Atherosclerosis* 166 (2003): 23–30.

53. K. F. Santos, T. T. Oliveira, T. J. Nagem, A. S. Pinto, and M. G. Oliveira, "Hypolipidaemic Effects of Naringenin, Rutin, Nicotinic Acid and Their Associations," *Pharmacological Research* 40 (1999): 493–496.

54. D. Rein, T. G. Paglieroni, T. Wun, D.A. Pearson, H. H. Schmitz, R. Gosselin, C. and L. Keen, "Cocoa Inhibits Platelet Activation and Function," *American Journal of Clinical Nutrition* 72 (2000): 30–35.

55. S. J. Duffy, J. F. Keaney, Jr, M. Holbrook, N. Gokce, P. L. Swerdloff, B. Frei, and J. A. Vita, "Short- and Long-term Black Tea Consumption Reverses Endothelial

Dysfunction in Patients with Coronary Artery Disease," *Circulation* 104 (2001): 151–156.

56. I. C. W. Arts and P. C. H. Hollman, "Polyphenols and Disease Risk in Epidemiologic Studies," *American Journal of Clinical Nutrition* 81 (2005): 317S–325S.

57. I. C. Arts, P. C. Hollman, E. J. Feskens, H. B. Bueno de Mesquita, and D. Kromhout, "Catechin Intake Might Explain the Inverse Relation between Tea Consumption and Ischemic Heart Disease: The Zutphen Elderly Study," *American Journal of Clinical Nutrition* 74 (2001): 227–232.

58. L. Yochum, L. H. Kushi, K. Meyer and A. R. Folsom, "Dietary Flavonoid Intake and Risk of Cardiovascular Disease in Postmenopausal Women," *American Journal of Epidemiology* 149 (1999): 943–949.

59. E. B. Rimm, M. B. Katan, A. Ascherio, M. J. Stampfer, and W. C. Willett, "Relation between Intake of Flavonoids and Risk for Coronary Heart Disease in Male Health Professionals," *Annals of Internal Medicine* 125 (1996): 384–389.

60. J. Lin, K. M. Rexrode, F. Hu, C. M. Albert, C. U. Chae, E. B. Rimm, M. J. Stampfer, and J. E. Manson, "Dietary Intakes of Flavonols and Flavones and Coronary Heart Disease in US Women," *American Journal of Epidemiology* 165, no. 11 (2007): 1305–1313.

61. P. Knekt, J. Kumpulainen, R. Jarvinen, H. Rissanen, M. Heliövaara, A. Reunanen, T. Hakulinen, and A. Aromaa, "Flavonoid Intake and Risk of Chronic Diseases," *American Journal of Clinical Nutrition* 76 (2002): 560–568.

62. C. S. Yang, J. M. Landau, M. T. Huang, and H. L. Newmark, "Inhibition of Carcinogenesis by Dietary Polyphenolic Compounds," *Annual Review of Nutrition* 21 (2001): 381–406.

63. M. Suschetet, M. H. Siess, A. M. Le Bon, and M. C. Canivenc-Lavier, "Anticarcinogenic Properties of Some Flavonoids," in: *Polyphenols* 96 (1997): 165–204. Vercauteren, J. and Triaud J. Cheze (eds). Paris, INRA Editions.

64. M. Barthelman, W. B. Bair, K. K. Strickland, W. Chen, B. N. Timmermann, S. Valcic, Z. Dong, and G. T. Bowden, "(-)-Epigallocatechin-3-Gallate Inhibition of Ultraviolet B-induced AP-1 Activity," *Carcinogenesis* 19 (1998): 2201–2204.

65. R. P. Webster, M. D. Gawde, and R. K. Bhattacharya, "Protective Effect of Rutin, a Flavonol Glycoside, on the Carcinogen-induced DNA Damage and Repair Enzymes in Rats," *Cancer Letters* 109 (1996): 185–191.

66. I. C. W. Arts and P. C. H. Hollman, "Polyphenols and Disease Risk in Epidemiologic Studies," *American Journal of Clinical Nutrition* 81 (2005): 317S–325S.

67. P. Knekt, J. Kumpulainen, R. Jarvinen, H. Rissanen, M. Heliövaara, A. Reunanen, T. Hakulinen, and A. Aromaa, "Flavonoid Intake and Risk of Chronic Diseases," *American Journal of Clinical Nutrition* 76 (2002): 560–568.

68. I. C. W. Arts, D. R. Jacobs, Jr. M. Gross, L. J. Harnack, and A. R. Folsom, "Dietary Catechins and Cancer Incidence among Postmenopausal Women: The Iowa Women's Health Study (United States)," *Cancer Causes Control* 13 (2002): 737–382.

69. Y. Levites, T. Amit, M. B. Youdim, and S. Mandel, "Involvement of Protein Kinase C Activation and Cell Survival/Cell Cycle Genes in Green Tea Polyphenol, (-)-Epigallocatechin-3-Gallate Neuroprotective Action. Attentuation of 6-Hydroxydopamine (6-OHDA)-Induced Nuclear Factor-Kappab (NF-Kappab) Activation and Cell Death by Tea Extracts in Neuronal Cultures," *Journal of Biological Chemistry* 63 (2002): 21–29.

70. W. Mullen, B. A. Graf, S. T. Caldwell, R. C. Hartley, G. G. Duthie, C. A. Edwards, M. E. Lean, and A. Crozier, "Determination of Flavonol Metabolites in Plasma and Tissues of Rats by HPLC-radiocounting and Tandem Mass Spectrometry Following Oral Ingestion Of [2(14)C]Quercetin-4'-Glucoside," *Journal of Agricultural and Food Chemistry* 50 (2002): 6902–6909.

71. J. A. Joseph, B. Shukitt-Hale, N. A. Denisova, D. Bielinski, A. Martin, J. J. McEwen, and P. C. Bickford, "Reversals of Age-related Declines in Neuronal Singal Transduction, Cognitive, and Motor Behavioral Deficits with Blueberry, Spinach, or Strawberry Dietary Supplementation," *Journal of Neuroscience* (1999): 8114–8121.

72. G. Y. Sun, J. Xia, B. Draczynska-Lusiak, A. Simonyi, and A. Y. Sun, "Grape Polyphenols Protect Neurodegenerative Changes Induced by Chronic Ethanol Administration," *Neuroreport* 10 (1999): 93–96.

73. Y. Levites, O. Weinreb, G. Maor, M. B. Youdim, and S. Mandel, "Green Tea Polyphenol (-)-Epigallocatechin-2-Gallate Prevents N-Methyl-4-Phenyl-1,2,3,6-Tetrahydropyridine-induced Dopaminergic Neurodegeneration," *Journal of Neurochemistry* 78 (2001): 1073–1082.

74. D. Commenges, V. Scotet, S. Renaud, H. Jacqmin-Gadda, P. Barberger-Gateau P, and J. F. Dartigues, "Intake of Flavonoids and Risk of Dementia," *European Journal of Epidemiology* 16 (2000): 357–363.

75. H. M. Evans and K. S Bishop, "On the Existence of a Hitherto Unrecognized Dietary Factor Essential for Reproduction," *Science* 56 (1922): 650–651.

76. H. A. Mattill and R. E. Conklin, "The Nutritive Properties of Milk, with special reference to Reproduction in the Albino Rat," *Journal of Biological Chemistry* 44 (1920): 137–158; T. B. Osborne and L. B. Mendel, "The Nutritive Value of Yeast Protein," *Journal of Biological Chemistry* 38 (1919): 223–227.

77. H. M. Evans and K. S. Bishop, "The Production of Sterility with Nutritional Regimes Adequate for Growths and Its Cure with Other foodstuffs," *Journal of Metabolic Research* 3 (1923): 233–316.

78. B. Sure, "Dietary Requirements for Reproduction. II The Existence of a Specific Vitamin for Reproduction," *Journal of Biological Chemistry* 58 (1924): 693–709.

79. H. S. Olcott and H. A. Mattill, "The Unsaponifiable Lipids of Lettuce. II Fractionation," *Journal of Biological Chemistry* 93 (1931): 59–64.

80. H. M. Evans, O. M. Emerson, and G. A. Emerson, "The Isolation from Wheat Germ Oil Ofan Alcohol, A-Tocopherol, Having the Properties of Vitamin E," *Journal of Biological Chemistry* 113 (1936): 319–332.

81. E. Fernholz, "On the Constitution of A-Tocopherol," *Journal of the American Chemical Society* 60 (1938): 700–705.

82. P. Karrer, H. Fritzsche, B. H. Ringier, and H. Salomon, "A-Tocopherol," *Helvitica Chimica Acta* 21 (1938): 520–525.

83. L. I. Filer, Jr., R. E. Rumery, and K. E. Mason, "Specific Unsaturated Fatty Acids in the Production of Acid-fast Pigment in the Vitamin E-deficient Rat and the Protective Action of Tocopherols," *Transactions of the First Conference on Biological Antioxidants*, New York: Josiah Macy, Jr. Foundation, 1946, 67–76; K. E.Mason and L. I. Filer, Jr., "Interrelationships of Dietary Fat and Tocopherols," *Journal of the American Oil Chemists Society* 24 (1947): 240–242.

84. K. E. Mason and I. R. Telford, "Some Manifestations of Vitamin E Deficiency in the Monkey," *Archives of Pathology* 43 (1947): 363–373; L. J. Filer, R. E. Rumery, Y. U. PNG, and K.E. Mason, "Studies on Vitamin E Deficiency in the Monkey," *Annals of the New York Academy of Sciences* 52 (1949): 284–289.

85. W. A. Pryor, "Vitamin E and Heart Disease: Basic Science to Clinical Intervention Trials," *Free Radical Biology & Medicine* 28, no. 1 (January 1, 2000): 141–164.

86. I. Jialal and C. J. Fuller, "Effect of Vitamin E, Vitamin C and Beta-carotene on LDL Oxidation and Atherosclerosis," *Canadian Journal of Cardiology* 11, Suppl. G (1995): 97G–103G.

87. M. G. Traber, "Heart Disease and Single-vitamin Supplementation," *American Journal of Clinical Nutrition* 85, no. 1 (2007): 293S–299S.

88. A. B. Weitberg and D. Corvese, "Effect of Vitamin E and Beta-carotene on DNA Strand Breakage Induced by Tobacco-specific Nitrosamines and Stimulated Human Phagocytes," *Journal of Experimental and Clinical Cancer Research* 16 (1997): 11–14.

89. M. Horwitt, W. Elliott, P. Kanjananggulpan, and C. Fitch, "Serum concentrations of Alpha-tocopherol after Ingestion of Various Vitamin E Preparations," *American Journal of Clinical Nutrition* 40, no. 2 (1984): 240–245.

90. Food and Nutrition Board, Institute of Medicine of the National Academies, *Dietary Reference Intakes for Vitamin C, Vitamin E, Selenium, and Carotenoids*, Washington, DC: National Academy Press, 2000.

91. M. Meydani, "Effect of Functional Food Ingredients: Vitamin E Modulation of Cardiovascular Diseases and Immune Function in Elderly," *American Journal of Clinical Nutrition* 71, no. 6 (2000): 1665–1668.

92. E. Miller, R. Pastor-Barriuso, D. Dalal, R. Riemersma, L. Appel, and E. Guallar, "Meta-analysis: High-dosage Vitamin E Supplementation May Increase All-cause Mortality," *Annals of Internal Medicine* 142, no. 1 (2005): 37–46.

93. P. G. Shekelle, S. C. Morton, L. K. Jungvig, J. Udani, M. Spar, W. Tu, M. J Suttorp, I. Coulter, S. J. Newberry, and M. Hardy, "Effect of Supplemental Vitamin E for the Prevention and Treatment of Cardiovascular Disease," *Journal of General Internal Medicine* 19, no. 4 (2004): 380–389; D. P. Vivekananthan, M. S. Penn, S. K. Sapp, A. Hsu, and E. J. Topol, "Use of Antioxidant Vitamins for the Prevention of Cardiovascular Disease: Meta-analysis of Randomised Trials," *Lancet* 364, no. 9374 (2003): 2017–2023; R. S. Eidelman, D. Hollak, P. R. Hebert, G. A. Lamas, and C. H. Hennekens, "Randomized Trials of Vitamin E in the Treatment and Prevention of Cardiovascular Disease," *Archives of Internal Medicine* 164, no. 14 (2004): 1552–1556.

94. J. N. Hathcock, D. Hollar, P. R. Hebert, G. A. Lamas, and C. H. Hennekens, "Vitamins E and C are Safe across a Broad Range of Intakes," *American Journal of Clinical Nutrition* 51, no. 4 (2005): 736–745.

95. E. M. Lonn and S. Yusuf, "Is There a Role for Antioxidant Vitamins in the Prevention of Cardiovascular Diseases? An Update on Epidemiological and Clinical Trials Data," *Canadian Journal of Cardiology* 13 (1997): 957–965.

96. M. J. Stampfer, C. H. Hennekens, J. E. Manson, G. A. Colditz, B. Rosner, and W. C. Willett, "Vitamin E Consumption and the Risk of Coronary Disease in Women," *New England Journal of Medicine* 328 (1993): 1444–1449.

97. P. Knekt., A. Reunanen, R. Jarvinen, R. Seppanen, M. Heliovaara, and A. Aromaa, "Antioxidant Vitamin Intake and Coronary Mortality in a Longitudinal Population Study," *American Journal of Epidemiology* 139 (1994): 1180–1189.

98. D. D. Waters, E. L. Alderman, J. Hsia, B. V. Howard, F. R. Cobb, W. J. Rogers, P. Ouyang, P. Thompson, J. C. Tardif, L. Higginson, V. Bittner, M. Steffes, D. J. Gordon, M. Proschan, N. Younes, and J. I. Verter, "Effects of Hormone Replacement Therapy and Antioxidant Vitamin Supplements on Coronary Atherosclerosis in Postmenopausal Women: A Randomized Controlled Trial," *Journal of the American Medical Association* 288 (2002): 2432–2440.

99. The Heart Outcomes Prevention Evaluation Study Investigators, "Vitamin E Supplementation and Cardiovascular Events in High-risk Patients," *New England Journal of Medicine* 342 (2000): 154–160.

100. J. Virtamo, P. Pietinen, J. K. Huttunen, P. Korhonen, N. Malila, M. J. Virtanen, D. Albanes, P. R. Taylor, and P. Albert, "ATBC Study Group. Incidence of Cancer and Mortality Following Alpha-tocopherol and Beta-carotene Supplementation: A Postintervention Follow-up," *JAMA* 290, no. 4 (July 2003): 476–485.

101. G. G. Kimmick, R. A. Bell, and R. M. Bostick, "Vitamin E and Breast Cancer: A Review," *Nutrition & Cancer* 27, no. 2 (1997): 109–117; R. Jarvinen, P. Knekt, R. Seppanen, and L. Teppo, "Diet and Breast Cancer Risk in a Cohort of Finnish Women," *Cancer Letters* 114, no. 1–2 (March 19, 1997): 251–253.

102. K. Helzlsouer, H. Huang, A. Alberg, S. Hoffman, A. Burke, E. Norkus, J. Morris, and G. Comstock, "Association between Alpha-tocopherol, Gamma-tocopherol, Selenium, and Subsequent Prostate Cancer," *Journal of the National Cancer Institute* 92, no. 24 (2000): 2018–2023.

103. S. Graham, M. Sielezny, J. Marshall, R. Priore, J. Freudenheim, J. Brasure, B. Haughey, P. Nasca, and M. Zdeb, "Diet in the Epidemiology of Postmenopausal Breast Cancer in the New York State Cohort," *American Journal of Epidemiology* 136 (1992): 3127–3137.

104. R. M. Bostick, J. D. Potter, D. R. McKenzie, T. A. Sellers, L. H. Kushi, K. A. Steinmetz, and A. R. Folsom, "Reduced Risk of Colon Cancer with High Intakes of Vitamin E: The Iowa Women's Health Study," *Cancer Research* 15 (1993): 4230–4237.

105. K. Wu, W. C. Willett, J. M. Chan, C. S. Fuchs, G. A. Colditz, E. B. Rimm, and E. L. Giovannucci, "A Prospective Study on Supplemental Vitamin E Intake and Risk of Colon Cancer in Women and Men," *Cancer Epidemiology Biomarkers and Prevention* 11 (2002): 1298–1304.

106. E. J. Jacobs, A. K. Henion, P. J Briggs, C. J. Connell, M. L. McCullough, C. R. Jonas, C. Rodriguez, E. E. Calle, and M. J. Thun, "Vitamin C and Vitamin E Supplement Use and Bladder Cancer Mortality in a Large Cohort of U.S. Men and Women," *American Journal of Epidemiology* 156 (2002): 1002–1010.

107. V. A. Kirsh, R. B. Hayes, S. T. Mayne, N. Chatterjee, A. F. Subar, L. B. Dixon, D. Albanes, G. L. Andriole, D. A. Urban, and U. Peters; PLCO Trial, "Supplemental and Dietary Vitamin E, Beta-carotene, and Vitamin C Intakes and Prostate Cancer Risk," *Journal of the National Cancer Institute* 98, no. 4 (February 15, 2006): 245–254.

108. H. Hemila et al., "The Effect of Vitamin E on Common Cold Incidence is Modified by Age, Smoking and Residential Neighborhood," *American Journal of Clinical Nutrition* 25, no. 4 (2006): 332–339.

109. M. C. Leske, L. T. Chylack, Jr., Q. He, S. Y. Wu, E. Schoenfeld, J. Friend, and J. Wolfe, "Antioxidant Vitamins and Nuclear Opacities: The Longitudinal Study of Cataract," *Ophthalmology* 105 (1998): 831–836.

110. J. M. Teikari, J. Virtamo, M. Rautalahti, J. Palmgren, K. Liesto, and O. P. Heinonen, "Long-term Supplementation with Alpha-tocopherol and Beta-carotene and Age-related Cataract," *Acta Ophthalmologica Scandinavica* 75 (1997): 634–640.

111. Age-Related Eye Disease Study Research Group, "Risk Factors Associated with Age-related Macular Degeneration; a Case-control Study in the Age-related Eye Disease," *Ophthalmology* 107 (2000): 2224–2232.

112. Age-Related Eye Disease Study Research Group, "A Randomized, Placebo-controlled, Clinical Trial of High-dose Supplementation with Vitamins C and

E, Beta-carotene, and Zinc for Age-related Macular Degeneration and Vision Loss," AREDS Report No. 8. *Archives of Ophthalmology* 119 (2001a): 1417–1436.

113. H. R. Taylor, G. Tikellis, L. D. Robman, C. A. McCarty, and J. J. McNeil, "Vitamin E Supplementation and Age-related Maculopathy," *Investigative Ophthalmology and Visual Science* 42 (2001): S311.

114. J. H. Kang, N. Cook, J. Manson, J. E. Buring, and F. Grodstein, "A Randomized Trial of Vitamin E Supplementation and Cognitive Function in Women," *Archives of Internal Medicine* 166 (2006): 2462–2468.

115. N. I. Krinsky and E. J. Johnson, "Carotenoid Actions and Their Relation to Health and Disease," *Molecular Aspects of Medicine* 26, no. 6 (December 2005): 459–516.

116. J. M. Holden, A. L. Eldridge, G. R. Beecher, M. Buzzard, S. Bhagwat, C. Davis, L. W. Douglass, S. Gebhardt, D. Haytowitz, and S. Schake, "Carotenoid Content of U.S. Foods: An Update of the Database," *Journal of Food Composition and Analysis* 12 (1999): 69–196.

117. M. Mozaffarieh, S. Sacu, and A. Wedrich, "The Role of the Carotenoids, Lutein and Zeaxanthin, in Protecting against Age-related Macular Degeneration: A Review based on Controversial Evidence," *Nutrition Journal* 2 (2003): 20

118. A. J. Young and G. M. Lowe, "Antioxidant and Prooxidant Properties of Carotenoids," *Archives of Biochemistry and Biophysics* 385 (2001): 20–27.

119. N. I. Krinsky, "Carotenoids and Oxidative Stress," in R. G. Cutler and H. Rodriguez (eds), *Oxidative Stress and Aging: Advances in Basic Science, Diagnostics, and Intervention*, New York: World Scientific Publishing Co., 2003, 598–611.

120. C. Rice-Evans, J. Sampson, P. M. Bramley, and D. E. Holloway, "Why Do We Expect Carotenoids to be Antioxidants In Vivo," *Free Radical Research* 26 (1997): 381–398.

121. C. S. Foote and R. W. Denny, "Chemistry of Singlet Oxygen. VIII. Quenching by B-Carotene," *Journal of the American Chemical Society* 90 (1968): 6233–6235.

122. K. L. Carpenter, C. van der Veen, R. Hird, I. F. Dennis, T. Ding, and M. J. Mitchinson, "The Carotenoids Beta-carotene, Canthaxanthin and Zeaxanthin Inhibit Macrophage-mediated LDL Oxidation." *FEBS Letter* 401 (1997): 262–266.

123. T. R. Dugas, D. W. Morel, and E. H. Harrison, "Impact of LDL Carotenoid and Alpha-tocopherol Content on LDL Oxidation by Endothelial Cells in Culture," *Journal of Lipid Research* 39 (1998): 999–1007.

124. A. J. A. Wright, S. Southon, M. Chopra, A. Meyer-Wenger, U. Moser, F. Granado, B. Olmedilla, B. Corridan, I. Hinninger, A.-M. Roussel, H. van den Berg, and D. I. Thurnham, "Comparison of LDL Fatty Acid and Carotenoid Concentrations and Oxidative Resistance of LDL in Volunteers from countries with Different Rates of Cardiovascular Disease," *British Journal of Nutrition* 87 (2002): 21–29.

125. C. M. Lee, A. C. Boileau, T. W. Boileau, A. W. Williams, K. S. Swanson, K. A. Heintz, and J. W. Erdman, Jr., "Review of Animal Models in Carotenoid Research," *Journal of Nutrition* 129 (1999): 2271–2277.

126. R. S. Parker, J. E. Swanson, C.-S. You, A. J. Edwards, and T. Huang, "Bioavailability of Carotenoids in Human Subjects," *Proceedings of the Nutrition Society* 58 (1999): 55–162.

127. C. Rice-Evans, J. Sampson, P. M. Bramley, and D. E. Holloway, "Why Do We Expect Carotenoids to Be Antioxidants In Vivo?" *Free Radical Research* 26 (1997): 381–398.

128. P. Palozza, "Prooxidant Actions of Carotenoids in Biologic Systems," *Nutrition Reviews* 56 (1998): 257–265.

129. X. D. Wang and R. M. Russell, "Procarcinogenic and Anticarcinogenic Effects of B-carotene," *Nutrition Reviews* 57 (1999): 263–272.

130. C. Liu, F. Lian, D. E. Smith, R. M. Russell, and X. D. Wang, "Lycopene Supplementation Inhibits Lung Squamous Metaplasia and Induces Apoptosis via Up-regulating Insulin-like Growth Factor-binding Protein 3 in Cigarette Smoke-exposed Ferrets," *Cancer Research* 63 (2003): 3138–3144.

131. S. T. Mayne, "Beta-carotene, Carotenoids, and Disease Prevention in Humans," *FASEB Journal* 10 (1996): 690–701.

132. Y. Ito, K. Suzuki, J. Ishii, H. Hishida, A. Tamakoshi, N. Hamajima, and K. Aoki, "A Population-based Follow-up Study on Mortality from Cancer or Cardiovascular Disease and Serum Carotenoids, Retinol and Tocopherols in Japanese Inhabitants," *Asian Pacific Journal of Cancer Prevention* 7, no. 4 (2006): 533–546.

133. B. Buijsse, E. J. Feskens, D. Schlettwein-Gsell, M. Kerry, F. J. Kok, D. Kromhout, and L. C. de Groot, "Plasma Carotene and Alpha-tocopherol in Relation to 10-y All-cause and Cause-specific Mortality in European Elderly: The Survey in Europe on Nutrition and the Elderly, a Concerted Action (SENECA)," *American Journal of Clinical Nutrition* 82, no. 4 (October 2005): 879–886.

134. Stavroula K. Osganian, Meir J. Stampfer, Eric Rimm, Donna Spiegelman, JoAnn E. Manson, and Walter C. Willett, "Dietary Carotenoids and Risk of Coronary Artery Disease in Women," *American Journal of Clinical Nutrition* 77 (June 2003): 390–1399.

135. D. L. Morris, S. B. Kritchevsky, and C. E. Davis, "Serum Carotenoids and Coronary Heart Disease: The Lipid Research Clinic's Coronary Primary Prevention Trial and Follow-up Study," *JAMA* 272, no. 18 (1994): 1439–1441.

136. R. Herrero, N. Potischman, L. A. Brinton, W. C. Reeves, M. M. Brenes, F. Tenorio, R. C. de Britton, and E. Gaitan, "A Case-control Study of Nutrient Status and Invasive Cervical Cancer. I. Dietary Indicators," *American Journal of Epidemiology* 134, no.11 (1991): 1335–1346.

137. C. H. Hennekens, J. E. Buring, J. E. Manson, M. Stampfer, B. Rosner, N. R. Cook, C. Belanger, F. LaMotte, J. M. Gaziano, P. M. Ridker, W. Willett, and R. Peto, "Lack of Effect of Long-term Supplementation with Beta Carotene on the Incidence of Malignant Neoplasms and Cardiovascular Disease," *New England Journal of Medicine* 334, no. 18 (1996): 1145–1149.

138. S. T. Mayne, D. T. Janerich, P. Greenwald, S. Chorost, C. Tucci, M. B. Zaman, M. R. Melamed, M. Kiely, and M. F. McKneally, "Dietary Beta Carotene and Lung Cancer Risk in U.S. Nonsmokers," *Journal of the National Cancer Institute* 86, no. 1 (1994): 33–38.

139. U. Peters, M. F. Leitzmann, N. Chatterjee, Y. Wang, D. Albanes, E. P. Gelmann, M. D. Friesen, E. Riboli, and R. B. Hayes, "Serum Lycopene, Other Carotenoids, and Prostate Cancer Risk: A Nested Case-control Study in the Prostate, Lung, Colorectal, and Ovarian Cancer Screening Trial," *Cancer Epidemiology, Biomarkers and Prevention* 16, no. 5 (2007): 962–968.

140. G. E. Goodman, M. D. Thornquist, J. Balmes, M. R. Cullen, F. L. Meyskens, Jr., G. S. Omenn, B. Valanis, and J. H. Williams, Jr., "The Beta-Carotene and Retinol Efficacy Trial: Incidence of Lung Cancer and Cardiovascular Disease Mortality during 6-year Follow-up after Stopping Beta-carotene and Retinol Supplements," *Journal of the National Cancer Institute* 96, no. 23 (2004): 1743–1750.

141. E. R. Greenberg, J. A. Baron, T. D. Tosteson, D. H. Freeman, Jr, G. J. Beck, J. H. Bond, T. A. Colacchio, J. A. Coller, H. D. Frankl, R. W. Haile, J. S. Mandel, D. W. Nierenberg, R. Rothstein, D. C. Snover, M. M. Stevens, R. W. Summers, R. U. van Stolk, for The Polyp Prevention Study Group, "A Clinical Trial of Antioxidant Vitamins to Prevent Colorectal Adenoma. Polyp Prevention Study Group," *New England Journal of Medicine* 331, no. 3 (1994): 141–147.

142. J. A. Baron, B. F. Cole, L. Mott, R. Haile, M. Grau, T. R. Church, G. J. Beck, and E. R. Greenberg, "Neoplastic and Antineoplastic Effects of Beta-carotene on Colorectal Adenoma Recurrence: Results of a Randomized Trial," *Journal of the National Cancer Institute* 95, no. 10 (2003): 717–722.

143. D. H. Holben and A. M. Smith, "The Diverse Role of Selenium within Seleno-proteins: A Review," *Journal of American Dietetic Association* 99 (1999): 836–843.

144. P. R. Larsen, T. F. Davies, and I. D. Hay, "The Thyroid Gland," in J. D. Wilson, D. W. Foster, H. M. Kronenberg, and P. R. Larsen (eds), *Williams Textbook of Endocrinology,* 9th ed., Philadelphia: W.B. Saunders Company, 1998, 389–515.

145. R. Shamberger, "Selenium and Heart Disease II: Selenium and Other Trace Element Intakes and Heart Disease in 25 Countries," in D. Hemphill (ed.), *Trace Substances in Environmental Health,* Columbia, MO: University of Missouri Press, 1978.

146. J. Salonen, G. Alfthan, J. Huttunen, J. Pikkarainen, and P. Puska, "Association between Cardiovascular Death and Myocardial Infarction and Serum Selenium in a Matched-pair Longitudinal Study," *Lancet* 2, no. 8291 (1982): 175–179; J. Virtamo, E. Valkeila, G. Alfthan, S. Punsar, J. Huttunen, and M. Karvonen, "Serum Selenium and the Risk of Coronary Heart Disease and Stroke," *American Journal of Epidemiology* 122 (1985): 276–282.

147. T. A. Miettinen, G. Alfthan, J. K. Huttunen, J. Pikkarainen, V. Naukkarinen, S. Mattila, and T. Kumlin, "Serum Selenium Concentration Related to Myocardial Infarction and Fatty Acid Content of Serum Lipids," *British Medical Journal* 287 (1983): 517–519; J. Ringstad and V. Fonnebo, "The Tromso Heart Study: Serum Selenium in a Low-risk Population for Cardiovascular Disease and Cancer and Matched Controls," *Annals of Clinical Research* 19 (1987): 351–354; S. Salvini, C. Hennekens, J. Morris, W. Willett, and M. Stampfer, "Plasma Levels of the Antioxidant Selenium and Risk of Myocardial Infarction among US Physicians," *American Journal of Cardiology* 76 (1995): 1218–1221.

148. J. Ringstad and V. Fonnebo, "The Tromso Heart Study: Serum Selenium in a Low-risk Population for Cardiovascular Disease and Cancer and Matched Controls," *Annals of Clinical Research* 19 (1987): 351–354.

149. S. A. Stanner, J. Hughes, C. N. M. Kelly, and J. Buttriss, "A Review of the Epidemiological Evidence for the 'Antioxidant Hypothesis,'" *Public Health Nutrition* 7 (2004): 407–422.

150. L. Clark, "The Epidemiology of Selenium and Cancer," *Federation Proceedings* 44 (1985): 2584–2589; P. Knekt, J. Marniemi, L. Teppo, M. Heliovaara, and A. Aromaa, "Is Low Selenium Status a Risk Factor for Lung Cancer?" *American Journal of Epidemiology* 148 (1998): 975–982.

151. R. Shamberger, E. Rukovena, A. Longfield, S. Tytko, S. Deodhar, and C. Willis, "Antioxidants and Cancer. I. Selenium in Blood of Normal and Cancer Patients," *Journal of National Cancer Institute* 50 (1973): 863–870.

152. P. Knekt, A. Aromaa, J. Maatela, G. Alfthan, R. K. Aaran, M. Hakama, T. Hakulinen, R. Peto, and L. Teppo, "Serum Selenium and Subsequent Risk of Cancer

among Finnish Men and Women," *Journal of National Cancer Institute* 82 (1990): 864–868.

153. F. Fernandez-Banares, E. Cabre, M. Esteve, M. D. Mingorance, A. Abad-Lacruz, M. Lachica, A. Gil, and M. A. Gassull, "Serum Selenium and Risk of Large Size Colorectal Adenomas in a Geographical Area with a Low Selenium Status," *American Journal of Gastroenterology* 97 (2002): 2103–2108.

154. K. Yoshizawa, W. C. Willett, S. J. Morris, M. J. Stampfer, D. Spiegelman, E. B. Rimm, and E. Giovannucci, "Study of Prediagnostic Selenium Level in Toenails and the Risk of Advanced Prostate Cancer," *Journal of National Cancer Institute* 90 (1998): 1219–1224.

155. W. Blot, J.-Y. Li, P. R. Taylor, W. Guo, S. Dawsey, G. Q. Wang, C. S. Yang, S. F. Zheng, M Gail, and G. Y. Li, Y. Yu, L. Buo-qi, J. Tangrea, Y. Sun, F. Liu, J. F. Fraumeni, Y.-H. Zhang, Jr., and B. Li, "Nutrition Intervention Trials in Linxian, China: Supplementation with Specific Vitamin/Mineral Combinations, Cancer Incidence, and Disease-specific Mortality in the General Population," *Journal of National Cancer Institute* 85 (1993): 1483–1492.

156. S. Yu, J. Zhu, and W. Li, "Protective Role of Selenium against Hepatitis B Virus and Primary Liver Cancer in Qidong," *Biological Trace Element Research* 56 (1997): 117–124.

157. M. A. Beck, "Selenium and Vitamin E Status: Impact on Viral Pathogenicity," *Journal of Nutrition* 137 (2007): 1338–1340.

158. L. C. Clark, G. F. Combs, Jr., B. W. Turnbull, E. H. Slate, D. K. Chalker, J. Chow, L. S. Davis, R. A. Glover, G. F. Graham, E. K. Gross, A. Krongrad, J. L. Lesher, H. K. Park, B. B. Sanders, C. L. Smith, and J. R. Taylor, "Effects of Selenium Supplementation for Cancer Prevention in Patients with Carcinoma of the Skin. A Randomized Controlled Trial. Nutritional Prevention of Cancer Study Group," *Journal of American Medical Association* 276 (1996): 1957–1963.

159. A. J. Duffield-Lillico, B. L. Dalkin, M. E. Reid, B. W. Turnbull, E. H. Slate, E. T. Jacobs, J. R. Marshall, L. C. Clark and Nutritional Prevention of Cancer Study Group, "Nutritional Prevention of Cancer Study Group. Selenium Supplementation, Baseline Plasma Selenium Status and Incidence of Prostate Cancer: An Analysis of the Complete Treatment Period of the Nutritional Prevention of Cancer Trial," *BJU International* 91 (2003): 608–612.

160. X. D. Wang and R. M. Russell, "Procarcinogenic and Anticarcinogenic Effects of Beta-carotene," *Nutrition Reviews* 57, no. 9 pt 1 (1999): 263–272.

161. G. Bjelakovic, D. Nikolova, L. L. Gluud, R. G. Simonetti, and C. Gluud, "Mortality in Randomized Trials of Antioxidant Supplements for Primary and Secondary Prevention: Systematic Review and Meta-analysis," *JAMA* 297, no. 8 (2007): 842–857.

162. E. R. Miller, R. Pastor-Barriuso, D. Dalal, R. A. Riemersma, L. J. Appel and E. Guallar, "Meta-analysis: High-Dosage Vitamin E Supplementation May Increase All-Cause Mortality," *Annals of Internal Medicine* 142 (2005): 37–46.

163. Office of Dietary Supplements, National Institutes of Health, http//dietary-supplements.info.nih.gov/index.asp (accessed May 30, 2007).

CHAPTER 5

1. Jennifer J. Otten, Jennifer P. Hellwig, and Linda D. Meyers, "Carotenoids," *Dietary Reference Intakes: The Essential Guide to Nutrient Requirements.* Washington, DC:

The National Academies Press, 2006, 211–217; Jane Higdon, "Carotenoids. Alpha-Carotene, Beta-Carotene, Beta-Cryptoxanthin, Lycopene, Lutein, and Zeaxanthin," The Linus Pauling Institute, 2005, http://lpi.oregonstate.edu/infocenter/phytochemicals/carotenoids (accessed March 26, 2007).

2. Otten et al., *Dietary Reference Intakes*, 215–216.

3. Ibid., 179.

4. Ibid., 213–216.

5. Higdon et al., "Carotenoids"; James A. Olson, Cheryl L. Rock, A. Catharine Ross, and Barbara A. Underwood, "Dietary Supplement Fact Sheet: Vitamin A and Carotenoids," Office of Dietary Supplements, National Institutes of Health, 2006, http://ods.od.nih.gov/factsheets/vitamina.asp (accessed April 24, 2007).

6. Otten et al., *Dietary Reference Intakes*, 171–181.

7. Ibid., 203–209.

8. Jane Higdon, "Vitamin C," The Linus Pauling Institute, 2006, http://lpi.oregonstate.edu/infocenter/vitamins/vitaminC/index.html (accessed April, 24 2007).

9. Otten et al., *Dietary Reference Intakes*, 208.

10. Ibid., 95–166.

11. Ibid., 206–207.

12. Ibid., 209–208.

13. Karen Collins, "How to Get More Cancer-fighting Nutrients," MSNBC, December 9, 2005, http://www.msnbc.msn.com/id/10281995 (accessed April 23, 2007).

14. Otten et al., *Dietary Reference Intake*, 239.

15. Sarah L. Zelinski, "Antioxidant May Have Adverse Effects in Head and Neck Cancer Patients," *Journal of the National Cancer Institute* 97, no. 7 (2005): 468–470, http://jnci.oxfordjournals.org/cgi/content/full/97/7/467-a (accessed April 23, 2007).

16. Charles Hennekens, Paul LaChance, Roger McDonald, and Maret Traber, "Vitamin E," Office of Dietary Supplements, National Institutes of Health, 2007, http://ods.od.nih.gov/factsheets/vitamine.asp (accessed April 24, 2007).

17. Ibid., 238.

18. Otten et al., *Dietary Reference Intakes*, 238–240.

19. Jed Fahey, Marianna Fordyce-Baum, Orville Levander, Keith West, and SedighehYamini, "Dietary Supplement Fact Sheet: Selenium," Office of Dietary Supplements, National Institutes of Health, 2004, http://ods.od.nih.gov/factsheets/selenium.asp (accessed April 24, 2007).

20. Food and Nutrition Board, Institute of Medicine of the National Academies, *Dietary Reference Intakes for Vitamin C, Vitamin E, Selenium, and Carotenoids.* Washington, DC: National Academy Press, 2000, 309.

21. Otten et al., *Dietary Reference Intakes*, 382–384.

22. Donald Buhler and Cristobal Miranda, "Antioxidant Activities of Flavonoids," The Linus Pauling Institute, 2000, http://lpi.oregonstate.edu/f-w00/flavonoid.html (accessed April 24, 2007).

23. Claudine Manach, Augustin Scalbert, Christine Morand, Christian Remesy, and Liliana Jimenez, "Polyphenols: Food Sources and Bioavailability," *American Journal of Clinical Nutrition* 79 (2004): 727–747, http://www.ajcn.org/cgi/reprint/79/5/727.pdf (accessed April 24, 2007).

24. Office of Dietary Supplements, "Facts about Dietary Supplements: Zinc," National Institutes of Health, 2002, http://dietary-supplements.info.nih.gov/factsheets/cc/zinc.html (accessed April 24, 2007).

25. Otten et al., *Dietary Reference Intakes*, 406.

26. Ibid., 410–411.

27. Jane Higdon, "Coenzyme Q10," The Linus Pauling Institute, 2007, http://lpi.oregonstate.edu/infocenter/othernuts/coq10/index.html (accessed April 24, 2007).

CHAPTER 6

1. Donald R. Davis, Melvin D. Epp, and Hugh D. Riordan, "Changes in USDA Food Composition Data for 43 Garden Crops, 1950 to 1999," *Journal of the American College of Nutrition* 23, no. 6 (2004): 669–682, http://www.jacn.org/cgi/content/abstract/23/6/669 (accessed April 29, 2007); Megan Carpenter, "Fruits, Veggies Not as Vitamin Rich as in Past, Says New Data," ABC News Internet Ventures (March 1, 2006), http://abcnews.go.com/Health/print?id=1671868 (accessed April 29, 2007).

2. D. K. Asami, Y.-J. Hong, D. M. Barrett, and A. E. Mitchell, "Comparison of the Total Phenolic and Ascorbic Acid Content of Freeze-Dried and Air-Dried Marionberry, Strawberry, and Corn Grown Using Conventional, Organic, and Sustainable Agricultural Practices," *Journal of Agriculture and Food Chemistry* 51, no. 5 (2003): 1237–1241.

3. V. Worthington, "Nutritional Quality of Organic Versus Conventional Fruits, Vegetables, and Grains," *The Journal of Alternative and Complementary Medicine* 7, no. 2 (April 2001): 161–173.

4. "Sprinkles Prove Effective in Controlling Anemia," *NutraUSAingredients.com*, March 26, 2003, http://www.nutraingredients-usa.com/news (accessed May 25, 2007).

5. Chris Woolston, "Do You Really Need to Know Your Antioxidant Level?" *Los Angeles Times*, March 5, 2007.

6. Marion Nestle, *Food Politics*, Berkeley, Los Angeles, London: University of California Press, 2002, 222–246.

7. Stephen Barrett, "How the Dietary Supplement Health and Education Act of 1994 Weakened the FDA," *Quackwatch*, February 2, 2007, http://www.quackwatch.org/02ConsumerProtection/dshea.html (accessed April 21, 2007).

8. Daron Watts, "Why NNFA Supports the AER Bill," *NNFA Today, Regulatory & Legislative News* 20, no. 6 (June 2006): 4–5, http://www.naturalproductsassoc.org/site/DocServer/June06.pdf?docID=1982 (accessed April 29, 2007).

9. Judy Foreman, "The Fading Allure of Vitamins," *Boston Globe*, May 14, 2007, http://www.boston.com/globe/health_science/articles/2007/05/14/the_fading_allure_of_vitamins?mode=PF (accessed May 14, 2007).

10. John Schmeltzer, "Kraft Eyes Profits in Health," *Chicago Tribune*, April 19, 2007, http://www.chicagotribune.com/business/chi-0704180612apr19,0,7866545, print.story?coll=chi-business-hed (accessed May 1, 2007).

11. Andrew Martin, "Want Vitamins and Minerals with That Soda?" *The New York Times*, March 14, 2007, http://content.hamptonroads.com/story.cfm?story=121056&ran=73351 (accessed May 15, 2007).

12. http://www.smartstart.com/ smart_start_antioxidants.shtml (accessed May 23, 2007).

13. Lorraine Heller, "Mars Moves to Capitalize on Growing Market for Healthy Snacking," *FoodNavigatorUSA.com*, October 10, 2006, http://www.foodnavigator-usa.com/news/printNewsBis.asp?id=7115 (accessed May 23, 2007); Cocoavia, "Three

Delicious Ways to Feel Good about Chocolate," Masterfoods, USA, http://www. cocoavia.be/en/products.asp (accessed May 23, 2007).

14. National Institutes of Health, "NIH State-of-the-Science Conference Statement on Multivitamin/Mineral Supplements and Chronic Disease Prevention," *Annals of Internal Medicine* 145 (2006): 364–371, http://consensus.nih.gov/2006/MVMFINAL080106.pdf (accessed January 12, 2007).

15. Elizabeth Frazao, "The American Diet: A Costly Health Problem–Moving Toward Healthier Diets," Agriculture Information Bulletin AIB-711, USDA (1995), http://findarticles.com/p/articles/mi_m3765/is_n1_v18/ai_19209855 (accessed May 23, 2007).

16. Kirstie Canene-Adams, Brian L. Lindshield, Shihua Wang, Elizabeth H. Jeffery, Steven K. Clinton, and John W. Erdman, Jr., "Combinations of Tomato and Broccoli Enhance Antitumor Activity in Dunning R3327-H Prostate Adenocarcinomas," *Cancer Research* 67, no. 2 (2007): 836–843, http://cancerres.aacrjournals.org/cgi/gca ?sendit=Get+All+checked+ . . . cer&FIRSTINDEX=0&HITS=10&RESULTFORMAT =&gca=canres%3B67%2F2%2F836 (accessed May 1, 2007).

17. Lydia A. Bazzano, "The High Cost of Not Consuming Fruits and Vegetables," *Journal of the American Dietetic Association* 106, no. 9 (September 2006): 1364–1366.

18. USDA, "Profiling Food Consumption in America," Agriculture Fact Book, 2001–2002, Chapter 2, http://www.usda.gov/factbook/chapter2.htm (accessed April 29, 2007).

19. Department of Health and Human Services and USDA, "Chapter 1. Background and Purpose of the Dietary Guidelines for Americans," *Dietary Guidelines for Americans 2005* (2007), http://www.health.gov/dietaryguidelines/dga2005/document/html/chapter1.htm (accessed May 25, 2007).

20. Department of Health and Human Services and USDA, "Chapter 2. Adequate Nutrients within Calorie Needs," *Dietary Guidelines for Americans 2005* (2007), http://www.health.gov/dietaryguidelines/dga2005/document/html/chapter1.htm (accessed May 25, 2007).

21. CDC, "About the National Fruit & Vegetable Program and Web Site," 2007, http://www.fruitsandveggiesmatter.gov/qa/index.html (accessed May 25, 2007).

22. Han-Yao Huang, Benjamin Caballero, Stephanie Chang, Anthony Alberg, Richard Semba, Christine Schneyer, Renee F. Wilson, Ting-Yuan Cheng, Gregory Prokopowicz, George J. Barnes, Jason Vassy, and Eric B. Bass, "Multivitamin/Mineral Supplements and Prevention of Chronic Disease," Agency for Healthcare Research and Quality, U.S. Department of Health and Human Services, AHRQ Publication No. 06-E012, Rockville, MD, May 2006, http://www.ahrq.gov/downloads/pub/evidence/pdf/multivit/multivit.pdf (accessed May 19, 2007).

23. Jacqueline Stenson, "A Vitamin a Day May Do More Harm than Good," *MSNBC.com*, January 19, 2007, http://www.msnbc.msn.com/id/16655168 (accessed January 19, 2007).

24. http://www.quotegarden.com/ayurveda.html (accessed April 11, 2007).

INDEX

Adequate intake (AI), 22, 23. *See also* Appendices A and B
Age-related macular degeneration (AMD), 56; AREDS study, 69–71, 78; vitamin E, 69
Alpha-carotene (α-carotene), 55, 71, 72, 73, 82, 83. *See also* Carotenoids; Vitamin A
Alpha-tocopherol (α-tocopherol), 38, 39, 55, 65, 66–67, 90, 92. *See also* Vitamin E
Alpha-Tocopherol Beta-Carotene Cancer Prevention Trial (ATBC), 55, 63, 69, 72, 73, 78, 82, 83
American Dietetic Association (ADA), 4; Nutrition and You Trends: 2000 study, 6
Anthocyanin, 21, 59, 96. *See also* Polyphenols
Antioxidants, 2, 9; carotenoid research, 71; co-enzyme Q10 research, 101–2; controversy, 49; definition, 20, 21, 31–32, 38; endogenous, 81; enzymes, 45; exogenous, 81; flavonoid research, 64–65; guidelines 107–16; polyphenol research, 96–99; selenium research, 76, 95; vitamin E research, 66; zinc research, 99–101. *See also* Carotenoids; Co-Enzyme Q10; Flavonoids; Polyphenols; Selenium; Vitamin A; Vitamin C; Vitamin E; Zinc

Ascorbate, ascorbic acid. *See* Vitamin C

Beta-carotene (β-carotene), 12, 19, 20, 38, 54, 55, 56, 57, 69, 71, 73, 77–78, 82, 83; carotenodermia, 83, 84, 106, 107. *See also* Carotenoids
Beta-Carotene and Retinol Efficacy Trial (CARET Study), 12, 55, 73–74, 78, 82, 83
Beta-cryptoxanthin (β-cryptoxanthin), 71, 82, 83. *See also* Carotenoids
Beta-monooxygenase (β-monooxygenase), 53

Cancer, ATBC and CARET studies, 55–56; carotenoids, 73–74; flavonoids, 63; Prevention of Cancer by Intervention with Selenium (PRECISE), 78; selenium, 76–78; vitamin E, 91, 96–97
Cardiovascular disease, vitamin C, 54; ATBC and CARET studies, 55; carotenoids, 72–74; flavonoids, 62–63; selenium, 76; vitamin E, 68
Carotenoids, 12, 20, 48, 57, 107; bioavailability, 83–84; cardiovascular disease, 72–74, 81; DRIs, 84, food sources, 95–87; vitamin A, 82–87; vitamin E, 65–68, 70–74
Catalase, 81
Catechins, 21, 59, 96. *See also* Polyphenols

Centers for Disease Control and
Prevention (CDC), 26, 55, 108,
112
Chocolate, 97. *See also* Polyphenols
Co-enzyme Q10 (Co-Q10), 81, 99–102;
food sources, 101
Commission on the Nomenclature of
Inorganic Chemistry, 34
Complementary and alternative medicine
(CAM), 1, 4; medical community,
9–10, 27
Consumerslab.com, 29, 105, 114
Continuing Survey of Food Intakes by
Individuals (CSFII), 6, 67; U.S. fruit
and vegetable intakes, 108

DASH Eating Plan, 109–12, 113–14
Dietary Guidelines for Americans, 2005,
109
Dietary Reference Intakes (DRIs), 12,
21–22; CoQ10, 102, 107;
polyphenols, 97; selenium, 95–96;
vitamin A and carotenoids, 84;
vitamin C, 89–90; vitamin E, 92–93.
See also Appendices A and B;
Estimated Average Requirement;
Recommended Dietary Allowance;
Recommended Nutrient Intake;
Tolerable Upper Intake Level
Dietary Supplement and Nonprescription
Drug Consumer Protection Act, 11,
12, 28, 105
Dietary Supplement Health and
Education Act of 1994 (DSHEA), 2,
10, 22, 26–28, 105
Dietary supplements, sales, 1–3;
adverse events, 27–29; consumer
characteristics, 6–9; definition,
25–26, 109; FTC and labeling
regulations, 26; recommendations, 13;
regulation and legislative history,
22–29; safety, 10–12

Ephedra, ephedrine, 27–29
Epicatechin, 21, 96. *See also* Polyphenols
Epigallocatechin-3-gallate (EGCG), 96.
See also Polyphenols
Estimated Average Requirement (EAR),
22, 23. *See also* Appendices A and B

Evolution of life, 41–46

Fenton reaction, 35, 42, 60. *See also*
Redox biology
Finnish Mobile Clinic Health
Examination Survey, 63, 77
5 A Day for Better Health Program, 108,
112. *See also* National Fruit and
Vegetable Program
Flavonoids, 12, 20, 31, 38, 58–65;
bioavailability, 61, 65; cancer, 63;
cardiovascular disease, 62–63;
chronic diseases, 61–62; flavanones,
flavones, flavonols, 59; neurological
disease, 63–65, 78–79, 96, 97, 103,
106. *See also* Polyphenols
Free radicals, definition, 32; free radical
theory of aging, 33–38; nomenclature,
34–41; 46, 47, 64; vitamin C, 88;
116. *See also* Redox biology
French Paradox, 97
Functional foods, definition, 2;
guidelines, 114–15; market sales, 2,
3, 10, 13, 31; marketing claims,
105–7, 109, 114; selenium, 94–95

Gallic acid, 39–40, 96. *See also*
Polyphenols
Gamma-tocopherol (γ-tocopherol), 92.
See also Vitamin E
Glutathione (GSH), oxidized glutathione
(GSSG), 39–40, 47–48, 61, 76, 81
Glutathione peroxidases (GPx;
glu-cys-gly), 47, 81; selenoproteins,
94. *See also* Selenium
GPx1, GPx2, GPx3, GPx4, 94. *See also*
Glutathione; Selenium
Green tea. *See* Polyphenols

Haber-Weiss reaction, 35. *See also* Redox
biology
Health and Human Services (HHS), 112
Health and Nutrition Examination
Survey (NHANES), history, 6; fruit and
vegetable intakes of Americans, 108;
NHANES I, 55; NHANES III, 67, 84,
89, 93, 95, 111; selenium, 95;
vitamin A, 84; vitamin E, 91; zinc,
100

Health of Americans, 3–4; *Healthy People 2010*, 108; *The State of Aging and Health in America 2007 Report*, 1, 108

The Health Professionals' Follow-up Study, 55, 62, 69

Heart Outcomes Prevention Evaluation (HOPE) Study, 68

History of nutrition, national studies, 5–9, 15–17; history of vitamin and mineral discoveries, 17–20

Institute of Medicine (IOM), 1, 2, 12, 20; Food and Nutrition Board, 20–21, 55, 57, 58, 67, 79, 80; nutrient intake recommendations, 103–14; vitamin A and carotenoids, 84; vitamin C, 88–89; vitamin E, 91, 93, 109

International Union of Pure and Applied Chemistry (IUPAC), 34

Iowa Women's Health Study, 62, 63, 69, 70

Iron heart theory, 54, 61

Isoflavones, 12, 21, 59. *See also* Polyphenols

Life stage groups, 23. *See also* Dietary Reference Intakes

Lignins, 21, 96. *See also* Polyphenols

Lind, Dr. James, 16, 52–53

Lutein, 20, 56, 71, 82, 83. *See also* Carotenoids

Lycopene, 20, 56, 73, 82; lycopenodermia, 83

Ma huang. *See* Ephedra

Multivitamin/multiminerals, 6, 7, 10, 11, 12, 77, 105, 109, 112–15

National Academy of Sciences, 1, 27; Panel on Dietary Antioxidants and Related Compounds of the IOM, 54, 55

National Cancer Institute (NCI), 55, 108

National Center for Complementary and Alternative Medicine (NCCAM), 12, 26, 64

National Fruit and Vegetable Program, 112

National health care costs in America, 3–4

National Health Examination Surveys (NHES), 6

National Health Interview Survey (NHIS), 5; selenium, 95; vitamin A, 84; vitamin E, 93

National Institute of Health (NIH), 1, 13, 26, 64, 107

NHANES. *See* Health and Nutrition Examination Survey

Nonprovitamin A carotenoids, 82. *See also* Carotenoids; Vitamin A

Nurses' Health Study, 55, 62, 69, 72

Nutraceuticals, definition, 2. *See also* Functional foods

Nutrient Content of USDA crops, 103–4; organic crops, 104

Nutrigenomics, 3

Nutrition and health surveys, history, 5–9

Office of Dietary Supplements (ODS), 26, 64, 80

Oxidative stress, 20, 49, 57, 78, 94

Physicians' Health Study, 56, 73

Phytochemicals, 20, 31, 38, 52, 112. *See also* Flavonoids; Polyphenols

Phytoestrogens. *See* Isoflavones

Polyphenols, 21, 31, 64, 81, 96–98; DRIs, 97; food sources, 97–98, 112. *See also* Anthocyanin; Catechins; Epicatechin; Epigallocatechin-3-Gallate; Flavonoids; Isoflavones; Lignins; Phytochemicals; Resveratrol; Stilbenes

Produce for Better Health Foundation, 108

Pro-oxidant, 32, 71; vitamin C, 88, 97

Provitamin A carotenoids, 81–84

Pseudoephedrine. *See* Ephedra

Pycnogenol, 64

Radicals, 33, 38, 47. *See also* Free Radicals

Reactive nitrogen species (RNS), 34, 38, 49, 61, 96

Reactive oxygen species (ROS), 34, 38, 41, 43, 48, 49; flavonoids, 60, 61, 96

Recommended Dietary Allowance (RDA), 21–22, 23; vitamin C, 57; vitamin E, 67. *See also* Appendices A and B

Recommended Nutrient Intake (RNI), 21–22. *See also* Appendices A and B

Red wine. *See* Resveratrol

Redox biology, 32–34. *See also* Antioxidants; Free radicals; Fenton reaction; Haber-Weiss reaction

Resveratrol, 21, 31

Retinal, retinoic acid, retinyl esters, 82. *See also* Vitamin A

Retinol, 55, 71, 82, 83, 84. *See also* Vitamin A

Selenate, selenite, selenocysteine, selenomethionine, 94. *See also* Selenium

Selenium, 12, 19, 20, 47, 57, 69, 74–78; bioavailability, 95; cancer, 76–78, 81, 93–96; cardiovascular disease, 76; food sources, 96

Selenoproteins, 93–94; thyroid metabolism, 94. *See also* Selenium

Stilbenes, 21, 31, 96. *See also* Polyphenols; Resveratrol

Superoxide dismutases (SOD), 33, 47, 81

Superoxide radical, 33, 46. *See also* Free radicals; Radicals

Tannins, 21, 96. *See also* Polyphenols

Thioredoxin reductase, 47. *See also* Selenium

Tocopherols, 66–67. *See also* Vitamin E

Tocotrienols, 66–67. *See also* Vitamin E

Tolerable Upper Intake Level (UL), 22, 23; selenium, 75, 79, 95, 112; vitamin C, 58, 89; vitamin E, 67–68, 91. *See also* Appendix B

Ubiquinone, 81, 101–2. *See also* Co-enzyme Q10

United States Department of Agriculture (USDA), 5, 95, 109, 112

United States Food and Drug Administration (FDA), 1, 3, 5, 10, 11, 24–29, 105

USDA Food Guide, 109, 110–14

Vitamin A, sales, 5, 12, 15, 17–20, 57, 70; carotenoids, 82–87; DRIs, 106, 109. *See also* Appendix B

Vitamin C (ascorbic acid), sales, 5, 6, 10, 12, 16, 17, 18, 20, 32, 38, 39, 40, 48, 52–58; bioavailability, 89; flavonoids, 60, 61, 68, 70, 72, 73, 74, 77–80, 81, 88–90; food sources, 90; selenium, 94, 97, 103, 104, 106, 107, 109

Vitamin E (α-tocopherol), sales, 5, 6, 9, 10, 12, 18, 20, 38, 39, 40, 48, 51, 54, 55, 56, 57, 61; bioavailability, 92–93; cancer, 69; cardiovascular, 68; carotenoids, 65–68; flavonoids, 97, 103, 106, 107, 109, 112; food sources, 92; neurological, 70, 73, 74, 77–79, 81, 90–93; RDA, 67; vision, 69–70

Vitamin K, 18; vitamin E, 91

Vitamin P, 21, 60

Women's Angiographic Vitamin and Estrogen (WAVE) trial, 68

World Health Organization (WHO), 1

Xenobiotic: definition, 35; metabolism, 37

Zeaxanthin, 71, 82, 83. *See also* Carotenoids

Zinc, 12, 70, 77, 99–101; bioavailability, 99; food sources, 100, 106. *See also* Appendix A

Zutphen Elderly Study, 62

About the Authors

PAUL E. MILBURY is a scientist at the Jean Mayer USDA Human Nutrition Research Center on Aging at Tufts University. His work is focused on determining dietary antioxidant bioavailability and effectiveness of nutrients in treating aging-related disorders. Before joining Tufts, Milbury was a Harvard Research Fellow at Massachusetts General Hospital studying oxidative stress in neurodegenerative disorders. He also served an 8-year tenure in the Long Range Research Lab at ESA, Inc., involved in a study of degenerative disorders funded by National Institute of Aging grants. Milbury holds a Ph.D. in animal and nutrition science, and degrees in animal science, cell biology, and chemistry, all from the University of New Hampshire.

ALICE C. RICHER is a registered, licensed dietician who has practiced in therapeutic, administrative, and education settings for more than 25 years. She is currently a consultant for nursing homes and an employee at Spaulding Rehabilitation Hospital Framingham Center, where she works with post-polio survivors, breast cancer survivors, and the professional soccer team, the New England Revolution. She trained at Beth Israel Hospital and earned her degrees at the University of Rhode Island and Boston College.